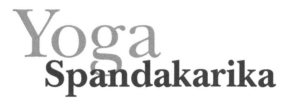

Yoga
Spandakarika

Yoga
Spandakarika

*The Sacred Texts at
the Origins of Tantra*

Daniel Odier

Translated from the French by Clare Frock

Inner Traditions
Rochester, Vermont

Inner Traditions
One Park Street
Rochester, Vermont 05767
www.InnerTraditions.com

Originally published in French under the title *L'Incendie du coeur: Le chant tantrique du frémissement* by Editions du Relié
First U.S. edition published in 2005 by Inner Traditions

Library of Congress Cataloging-in-Publication Data
Odier, Daniel, 1945-
  [Incendie du cœur. English]
  Yoga Spandakarika : the sacred texts at the origins of Tantra / Daniel Odier ; translated by Clare Frock.— 1st U.S. ed.
     p. cm.
  Translated from French and from Sanskrit.
  Originally published under title: L'incendie du cœur : le chant tantrique du frémissement. Relié.
  Includes the English translations of the Spandakaarikaa and of the Vijnaanabhairava.
  Includes bibliographical references.
  ISBN 978-1-59477-051-7
  1. Vasugupta. Spandakaarikaa. 2. Kashmir Saivism—Doctrines. I. Frock, Clare. II. Vasugupta. Spandakaarikaa. English. III. Tantras. Rudrayaamalatantra. Vijnaanabhairava. English. IV. Title.
  BL1281.1592.V38A2743613 2005
  294.5'95—dc22

                                                              2005001680

Printed and bound in the United States

15 14 13 12 11 10

Text design and layout by Virginia Scott Bowman
This book was typeset in New Baskerville, Cataneo, and Avenir as display typefaces

*My thanks go
to Anne Blum for her
work in transcribing the
oral commentaries*

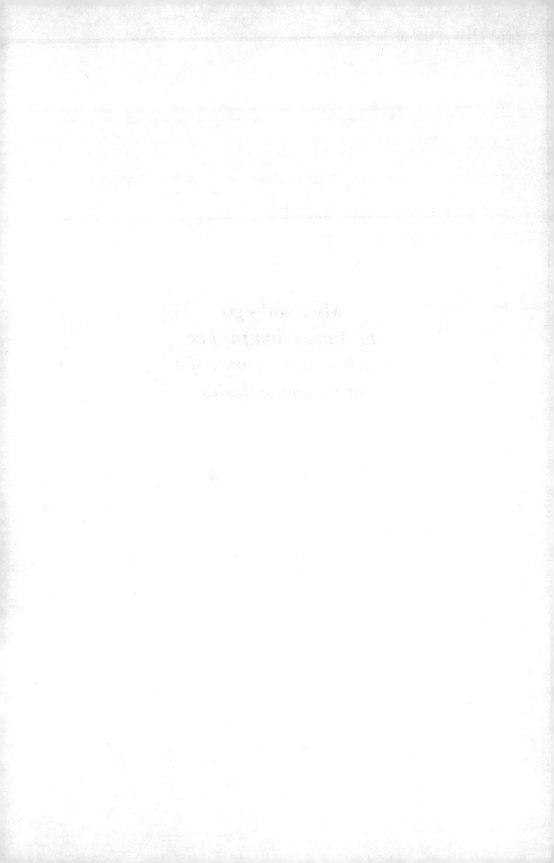

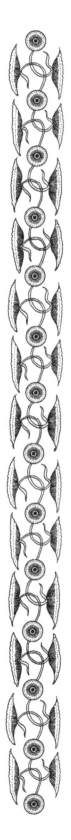

Contents

Preface
ix

The Ancient Text

Spandakarika:
The Tantric Song of the Sacred Tremor
2

The Commentary

First Flow (Stanzas 1–16):
The Instructions Concerning the Independent
Existence of the Self
16

Second Flow (Stanzas 17–27):
The Direct Perception of One's Own
Fundamental Nature
61

Third Flow (Stanzas 28–52):
The Universal Nature Reflected in the Power of
One's Own Nature
101

Conclusion:
Should One Practice Mahamudra?
140

Appendix 1:
Vijnanabhairava Tantra
147

Appendix 2:
The Natural Liberation through Naked Vision,
Identifying Intelligence
165

Notes
171

Preface

To my first meetings with the great Chinese, Tibetan, and Kashmiri masters, I owe the idea of the profound similarity between Ch'an,* Tantrism, Dzogchen, the Tibetan Mahamudra, and the original Mahamudra (that of Kashmiri Shaivism, a mystical movement linked to the teachings of the Mahasiddhas and to the Shaivism—Shiva worship—of the Indus Valley from six thousand years ago). Shiva is considered to be the creator of dance and yoga. His abode is Mount Kailash and he holds a trident, which symbolizes humankind as the divinity, the temple, and the worshipper—all united in the main branch of the trident.

In 1967, at the age of twenty-two, I arrived fresh from my readings in a shocking and marvelous India that would destroy, one by one, the ideas that I had established for myself regarding spirituality. Armed with a letter of recommendation that Arnaud Desjardins, the French reporter and spiritual teacher, had quite willingly written for me following my enthusiasm for his film series *Les Mystères des Tibétains,* I set out for Delhi. There, I met the director of the Tibetan Museum, who in

---

Translator's note: It may be helpful for readers to know that Ch'an, sometimes written "Chan," or "Tch'an," is Chinese Zen.

turn sent me to Kalimpong to meet the most prominent leader of the Nyingmapas, Dudjom Rinpoche. As chance (a word cursed by spiritualists) would have it, I stopped in front of a little house in which there lived a scholarly Chinese man by the name of Chien Ming Chen, author of some one hundred works unpublished in the West. This little bearded man, dressed in a worn, stain-spattered robe, radiated dazzling energy and overflowing joy. He served me tea before a yogini whose legs were spread open upon the space that he spent his days and his early mornings contemplating in unending ecstasy. He gave me as gifts more than twenty of his works, all of which I still have. Among these was a commentary on the *Vijnanabhairava Tantra*,[1] which it seems existed in Chinese, although it belonged originally to the Mahamudra of the siddhas in the Kashmiri Shaivism tradition.

This first meeting carried in seed form all of the future developments of my approach. Of all the works he gave me (which I carried about with me like a Himalayan mule), the *Vijnanabhairava Tantra* immediately and absolutely fascinated me. Chien Ming Chen was a follower of Ch'an but also of Dzogchen and Mahamudra. He had lived in his hermitage since 1947, without ever having gone outside of it. Curious souls who were now locally financing his printed publications had nevertheless found him. He fascinated both the masters of Hinayana Buddhism as well as those of the Mahayana and the Vajrayana, along with a few scientists and academics. I spent only a few hours in his company, but they were a determining factor in my opening to these various streams.

After having explained to me the ideal conditions for establishing a hermitage—conditions that I still remember and that governed my choice of place for my retreat in Tuscany—Chien Ming Chen, very modest man that he was, told me that he could not guide me on the path because his vow as a hermit constrained him to practicing only, and that he himself had not yet realized the ultimate fruit. He sent me to the great master and supreme leader of the Nyingmapa, Dudjom Rinpoche, the same man for whom the director of the Tibetan Museum of Delhi had written me a letter of recommendation.

With regret I left this remarkable man, and arrived that same day at a lovely Indian-style dwelling, a bungalow perched on a hill, where I was warmly welcomed by Dudjom Rinpoche's wife. During those golden days, the greatest masters were accessible with surprising ease. Few Westerners were seeking the dharma. Dudjom Rinpoche received me. He was a man who had an open gaze on the infinite, a perpetual smile on his face, great kindness, and an almost feminine gentleness allied with a gripping powerfulness. He had long hair and wore a Western shirt under his blue Tibetan robe. He granted all my requests. I had naively gotten it into my head to write a book on Tibetan painting with the support of the great art publisher Albert Skira, who had had me take a few courses on the photography of paintings and had then armed me with the appropriate materials. Dudjom Rinpoche had the thangkas (painted rolls) brought out from the temple and watched me photograph them, then informed me, with humor, that in order to penetrate their secrets, I would have to practice the path.

Troubles at the nearby Sino-Indian border were such that foreigners were not allowed to stay in Kalimpong for more than three days. The Indian authorities were being driven by an acute sense of spy mania, and for them, any foreigner was a potential informer of the Chinese. In the face of my enthusiasm, Dudjom Rinpoche gave me, over the course of each of my three days, the essence of the Dzogchen teachings; it would be thirty years before I understood how simple, vast, and direct his instruction had been. (Subsequently, I had the opportunity to meet with Kalu Rinpoche and to express my gratitude to him.) When I was leaving him, Dudjom Rinpoche gave me a letter of recommendation for one of his disciples who lived near Darjeeling: Chatral Rinpoche, also a great master of Dzogchen.

This meeting would turn out to be rough and upsetting. Having arrived at his place, I pushed open the door to a kind of hovel, and I found Chatral Rinpoche in contemplation, his gaze absolutely still and open straight in front of him. I remember a brazier, a thermos bottle on the table, and a calendar bearing the effigy of Gandhi. Standing before the master's silence, I took out the letter, which he did not read.

Abruptly and bluntly he asked me what I wanted. I made my request, trembling, so irrepressible and marvelous was the energy he emitted. He leaped up, caught me by the collar, and took me to a spot behind his lair, where there were six little retreat cells: loose boards and canvas roof. He opened a door and pushed me into one of these cubbyholes—which seemed more like a latrine than a place for contemplation—and said, "Are you ready to be in this cell for six years?" I came right back out, frightened by the cold, the rain, the fog, and the smallness of the place. He laughed and told me, "In that case, I can do nothing for you. Start by learning Tibetan."

I was quite happy at the idea of escaping from him. Just as I was leaving, he called out in a more friendly tone, "It's too bad. I only take six disciples at a time. There was an open space. You would have had the chance to attain awakening. But go down to Sonada; it's a few kilometers away. There you'll find your master."

I walked in the driving rain, thanking the gods for my having escaped this big-nosed typhoon. I imagined that the master awaiting me was going to be even more insane. I had the surprise of my life when I came into the room where a magnificent old man with eyes full of love was playing with a cat, balancing cans on its head, the cat looking at him as if hypnotized. After a brief conversation, Kalu Rinpoche told me right then and there that I could think of him as my master or as my mother. I chose the second option and relaxed completely in his presence, which emitted love like a soothing and nourishing elixir.

It was at Sonada that I undertook my long search, which would culminate much later with the transmission of the Mahamudra. I would discover, over the course of the weeks that followed, that Chatral and Kalu Rinpoche were very close. Chatral, at the wheel of his jeep (which he drove like a frenzied madman), visited Kalu quite frequently. He never missed the opportunity, while I was there, to make fun of this young, pretentious Westerner whose nose he had been so nice as to wipe.

In the years during which I followed the teachings of Kalu Rinpoche, I learned that he had realized the teachings of both the Dzogchen and the Mahamudra, the Direct Way, which many, many lives are not enough to reach. Kalu Rinpoche said:

> Mahamudra, the Great Symbol, or Dzogchen, the Great
> Perfection, are truly beyond the distinction between meditation
> and nonmeditation; thus it is not really right to name them in one
> way or another. Because they are the outcome of all the practices,
> one can conventionally say that they are the highest form of med-
> itation. Some people make a distinction between Dzogchen and
> Mahamudra, but that distinction is pointless because, fundamen-
> tally, these are two names for the same experience.[2]

I later learned that Kalu Rinpoche's father, a yogin and doctor,
had been a disciple of the famous Mipham Rinpoche, one of the great
Nyingmapa masters. Several learned masters of this school have con-
firmed that the Ch'an masters had had to retreat from Tibet after
their defeat at the infamous debate of Samye, but that the Nyingmapa
and the Kagyupa had preserved the essence of Ch'an under the names
of Dzogchen and Mahamudra. Many academics today explore this
route, and one may read with interest an article on the subject by
Guilaine Mala published in *Tch'an, Zen, racines et floraisons*.[3] Also
of interest are *Mahamudra: The Quintessence of Mind and
Meditation* by Takpo Tashi Namgyal,[4] and *A Spacious Path to
Freedom: Practical Instructions on the Union of Mahamudra and
Atiyoga* by Karma Chagmé,[5] both of which treat this question in
detail.

Once familiarized with Ch'an, I was not surprised when I noticed
that the teachings of the Bodhidharma[6] on the "two entrances" is systematically taken up again in the Dzogchen and the Mahamudra, and
that Dudjom Rinpoche and Kalu Rinpoche reserved a significant
amount of space for the subject in their teachings.[7]

When in 1975 I met the yogini Lalita Devi—who would become my
master and who would transmit to me the teachings of the Pratyabhijna
and Spanda of the Kashmiri Shaivism stream—I took it a step further
and grasped the impact of the Kashmiri siddhas on Tibetan Buddhism,

which, by the way, "Buddhafies" the siddhas to such a degree that Alain Daniélou would go on to write that "Tibetan Buddhism is Shaivism in disguise."[8] One of the most striking examples is Saraha's "Queen Doha," which includes the following stanzas:

A [Saivite] yogi in whom a [pseudoexistential] pristine
*   awareness [allegedly imparted to him by Siva himself] has*
*   come about, [and hence] in whom there is no fear,*
will, whilst wearing the insignia of Siva [as a charm], look for
*   a woman born in the outskirts.*

. . . Taking in her qualities he will [reciprocate by] offering his
*   pristine awareness,*
Reverberating within the intensity of immediate experience,
*   and,*
For the time being, he will take this pristine awareness—
*   heightened in its sensibility through Being's genuineness*
*   [operating in it], approximating in flavor,*
[Being's nothingness replete with everything in highest
*   perfection]—as the Mahamudra experience.*[9]

Scholars with Buddhist tendencies, uncomfortable with this passage, have it follow, or replace it with, similar verses—sometimes in parentheses, it is true—removing the allusion to Shaivism, just as they often delete, purely and simply, all allusion to Saraha's master, who was a Shaivite yogini.

It seems that in seventh- and eighth-century Kashmir, and even in later centuries, there reigned a great freedom of spirit and that the yogis and yoginis, when it was a matter of realizing the ultimate, hardly worried about the etiquette of the masters or about their belonging to one group or another. The great Abhinavagupta himself had many masters, some of whom were not Shaivite.

What I am proposing here is to rediscover this opening of mind by presenting the texts of Ch'an, Dzogchen, and the Mahamudras—Chinese, Tibetan, and Kashmiri—texts that only mystical experience can bring together. Several of these essential texts have been translated here into English for the first time. The teachings that follow come from the greatest masters of Kashmiri, Tibetan, and Indian Tantrism, but also from the great Ch'an masters who passed on the essence of Mahamudra. Their names are Abhinavagupta, Kshemaraja, Vasugupta, Kallata, Utpaladeva, Lalla, Savari, Virupa, Mazu, Niu-tou, Tao-sin, Dahui, Chen-houei, Foyan, Pao-tche, Machig, Yung Chia Hsuan Chueh, Jayratha, Padmasambhava, Vimalakirti, and Yuanwu.

I will add that, in 2002, to commemorate this union of the three streams that had the strongest impact upon me, I received, in Catalonia, the Ch'an ordination (Soto Zen lineage) from Master Kosen. What is a monk? According to Kosen, a monk is simply someone who is "in harmony with the cosmos." A lovely definition that spatializes, or brings space to, the vows by bringing them back to unending unity. Finally, in the spring of 2004 in China, I met the Grand Ch'an master Jing Hui, dharma heir of Xu Yun, better known in the United States as "Empty Cloud" (1839–1959),* who is recognized as the foremost Ch'an master of the twentieth century. My master Jing Hui gave me the Ch'an ordination in the Lin t'si and Caodong schools, as well as the permission to transmit the Zhao Zhou Ch'an spirit in the West.[10]

How to be in harmony with the cosmos? It seems that certain preliminaries are indispensable: Rid yourself of all beliefs; leave metaphysics to the sectarians of the absurd; understand that hope is fear gone bad; confront reality directly; stop upholding the romantic dream of realization; forget sentimental neurosis; play with your own limits; look at your confusion; confront life without the bric-a-brac of the religious and the spiritual—without, for all that, becoming a narrow-minded materialist who would make a new God out of rationalism; dare to be alone; do not oppose Essence against reality; give yourself over to the pleasures of pure subjectivity; understand that everything is real; and finally, one day, know exhilarating silence. Can one say that such a

---

*Translator's note: The dates are correct! XuYun, like Zhao Zhou, lived 120 years.

person is a mystic? According to the Shaivites, yes. According to the Ch'an masters, yes. According to the followers of Mahamudra, yes. In fact, all it takes is to say no to everything or to say yes to everything and to be an iconoclast who goes so far that he forgets the vehicle that brought him to this form of radical thinking. In short, it takes crazy wisdom.

The commentary on each stanza of the *Spandakarika,* or "Song of the Sacred Tremor," comprises three parts: the first is newly written by me; the second is a quotation from one of the great masters of the Mahamudra tradition; the third is the transcription of an oral teaching given during my seminar on this text. The commentary on each of the three "flows," or parts, of the *Spandakarika,* is followed by a great poem: the first by the yogini Machig Labdrön, the second by Padmasambhava, and the third by Tilopa. Two appendices follow: Appendix 1 is a translation of the complete text of the *Vijnanabhairava Tantra.* Appendix 2 is an alternate translation of the Padmasambhava poem that appears at the end of the second flow.

Today, having made Mahamudra my sole practice, in contemplation before the unbridled sea, I know that knowledge divides, and practice unites.

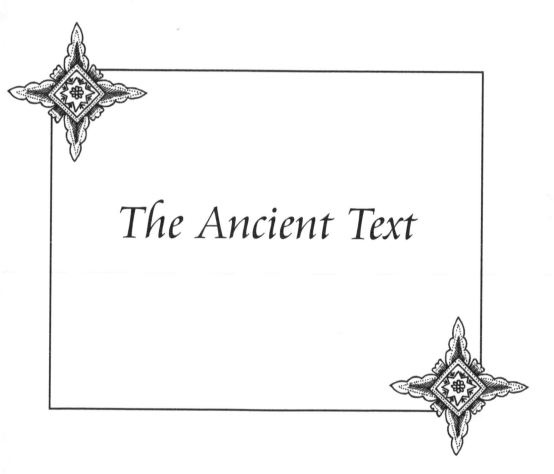

The Ancient Text

Spandakarika:
The Tantric Song
of the
Sacred Tremor

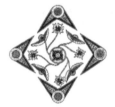

The *Spandakarika*, or "Song of the Sacred Tremor,"* is one of the essential texts of Kashmiri Shaivism. Having been revealed at the beginning of the ninth century by Shiva to Vasugupta, or to say it more directly, having gushed forth like a spring from Vasugupta's own heart, it presents the essence of the Tantras in fifty-two marvelously elliptical stanzas. They were written by Vasugupta himself or by his disciple

---

*Translator's note: The French word is *frémissement*, from the verb *frémir*, "to tremor, quiver, shudder, thrill, simmer (water)." Daniel Odier uses this word to convey the idea of the Sanskrit *spanda*, which has been translated variously as "vibration," "the divine pulsation," or "vibratory dynamism of the absolute consciousness." Here, the *sacred tremor* or *tremoring* will be used in the absence of a single English word that can adequately serve the rich meaning of the French and Sanskrit terms.

Kallata. Some say that Vasugupta received them in a dream while meditating in a cave in Mount Kailash, the mythical home of the trident-bearing god who gave birth to the sacred River Ganges. Ksemaraja, another important master of the tradition, who left a long commentary on the first stanza and to whom we owe the magnificent *Pratyabhijnahrdayam* or "Heart of Recognition," said that Vasugupta found them carved into a rock, and the faithful of today still revere the site.[1]

In his commentary, Ksemaraja stresses the fact that the "Song of the Sacred Tremor" is a presentation of Mahamudra, which would go on to become famous through the Tibetan lineage of transmission, and which is the ultimate teaching of the Kagyu school. Mahamudra is often translated as the "Great Seal," referring to the secret of this teaching and to the fact that it seals all that preceded it. But the Kashmiris translate it as the "Great Cosmic Movement" because its realization is linked to the yoga transmitted by Matsyendranath, who is at the source of the Kashmiri lineages. This siddha probably lived in Assam in the seventh century of the common era. Abhinavagupta, the great tenth-century philosopher and master, pays homage to Matsyendranath in his *Tantraloka,* which presents the sum of all knowledge on the Tantras.

This yoga, the teaching of which has almost completely disappeared, is very profound. It seems to have been the form that preceded hatha yoga. Its very simplicity is what makes it so difficult. The most ancient masters of the tradition had come to the realization that all is movement in the universe. They saw everything, including matter, as consciousness, and they invented a yoga that fit this realization. This sacred dance, called Tandava, is carried out in three phases: During the first stage, the body is released into space, the breath settles in, and the sacred tremoring of the organs is welcomed by consciousness, which allows this inner palpitation to become free and thus rejoins the limitless. Lalita Devi compared this sensation to the movements that moths flying within us might make. Little by little, the body lets itself go into an extremely slow, involuntary movement, where the limbs are carried by the breath in a circular unfolding.

In the second phase, the yogi lets his arms open out into space, the spinal column extremely supple, the eyelids slightly open, the tongue relaxed, the perineum open, the breath freed. The shoulder blades are open like wings and give balance to the body, which is normally drawn more toward the front. This whole yoga is practiced visualizing oneself naked, floating in midnight blue space.

In the third phase, the yogi gets up and allows his whole body to express the dance of Shiva in space. These movements look like a completely free kind of t'ai chi in which no movement is codified. The sequential linking of these movements make up the whole Kashmiri yoga such as I received its transmission from my master, yogini Lalita Devi.

This is an extremely subtle and difficult yoga that requires thousands of hours of practice. The advantage of this yoga is that it makes all other physical practice unnecessary. It can be seen in the sculptures of Tantric temples and in Tibetan statuary and paintings, which almost always represent the yogin, the yogini, and the divinities in this supple, lateral movement, and which one can imagine is omnidirectional. This tradition—so simple, so subtle—has gradually fallen into oblivion and been replaced by the more spectacular hatha yoga.

The *Spandakarika* presents the philosophy that was born of this practice, and all the yoga does is keep bringing us back to the source of this fundamental realization.

THE SONG OF THE SACRED TREMOR

1.
The venerated Shankari (Shakti), source of energy, opens her eyes and the universe is reabsorbed in pure consciousness; she closes them and the universe is manifested within her.

2.
The sacred tremor, the very place of creation and return, is completely limitless because its nature is formless.

3.
Even within duality, the tantrika goes straight to the nondual source, because pure subjectivity always resides immersed within his own nature.*

4.
All the relative notions tied to the ego rediscover their peaceful source deeply buried under all the different states.

5.
In the absolute sense, pleasure and suffering, subject and object, are nothing other than the space of profound consciousness.

---

*The pronoun *he* is used throughout in this translation in the interests of grammatical consistency.

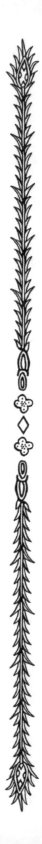

6., 7.

To grasp this fundamental truth is to see
absolute freedom everywhere. Thus, the
activity of the senses itself dwells in this
fundamental freedom and pours forth from it.

8.

Therefore, the person who rediscovers this
essential sacred tremor of consciousness
escapes the dim confusion of limited desire.

9.

Liberated in this way from the multiplicity of
impulses tied to the ego, he experiences the
supreme state.

10.

Then the heart realizes that the true innate
nature is both the universal agent and the
subjectivity that perceives the world. Thus
immersed in understanding, it knows and
acts according to its desire.

11.

How can this wonder-filled tantrika, who
always comes back to his own fundamental
nature as the source of all manifestation, be
subject to transmigration?

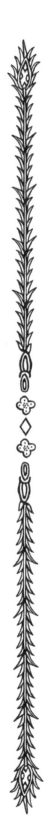

12.
If the void could be an object of
contemplation, where would the
consciousness that perceives it be?

13.
Therefore, consider contemplation of the
vacuity as an artifice of a nature analogous to
that of a profound absence from the world.

14., 15., 16.
Actor and action are united, but when action is
dissolved by abandoning the fruits of the act,
the very dynamic that is tied to the ego
exhausts itself, and the tantrika who is
absorbed in this profound contemplation
discovers the divine tremor liberated from its
ties to the ego. The profound nature of action
is thus revealed, and he who has interiorized
the movement of desire no longer knows
dissolution. He cannot cease to exist because
he has returned to the profound source.

17.
The awakened tantrika realizes this
continuous sacred tremor throughout the
three states.

18.
Shiva is then in loving union with Shakti in
the form of knowledge and its object,

whereas everywhere else he is manifested as
pure consciousness.

19.

The whole palette of the different kinds of
sacred tremoring finds its source in the
universal sacred tremor of consciousness,
and in this way reaches the person. How
could such a sacred tremoring limit the
tantrika?

20.

And yet, this sacred tremor itself causes
people who are subject to limited views to
become lost because, their intuition being
dissociated from the profound source, they
throw themselves into the whirlwind of
transmigration.

21.

The person who with fieriness tends toward
the profound sacred tremor reaches his true
nature even within activity.

22.

The profound and stable sacred tremor can
be reached in extreme states: anger, intense
joy, mental wandering, or the drive toward
survival.

23., 24.

When the tantrika gives himself over to
Shiva/Shakti, the sun and the moon come up
in the central channel.

25.

At that moment, when in the sky the sun and
the moon disappear, the awakened person
remains lucid, whereas the ordinary person
sinks into unconsciousness.

26., 27.

Mantras, when they are charged with the
power of the sacred tremor, accomplish their
function through the senses of the awakened
person. They become united with the mind
of the tantrika, who penetrates the nature of
Shiva/Shakti.

28., 29.

All things emerge from the individual
essence of the tantrika who recognizes
himself in Shiva/Shakti; everything in which
he takes pleasure is Shiva/Shakti. Thus, there
is no state that can be named that would not
be Shiva/Shakti.

30.

Always present to the reality that he perceives
as the play of his own nature, the tantrika is
liberated at the very heart of life.

31.

Through the intensity of objectless desire,
contemplation emerges in the heart of the
tantrika united to the profound sacred
tremor.

32.

This is the attainment of the supreme nectar,
the immortality of samadhi, which reveals to
the tantrika his own nature.

33., 34.

The ardor toward Shiva/Shakti that manifests
the universe allows the tantrika to be
fulfilled. Over the course of the dream, the
sun and the moon appear in his heart and all
his wishes are granted.

35.

But if he is not present, the tantrika will be
wronged by the play of manifestation, and
he will experience the illusory state of the
aspirant throughout waking and sleeping.

36., 37.

Just as an object that escapes attention is
more clearly perceived when we make the
effort to see it better from all angles, so the
supreme sacred tremor appears to the
tantrika when he ardently strives toward it. In

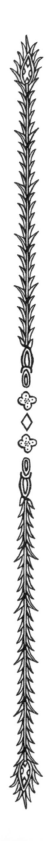

this way, everything is in tune with the
essence of his true nature.

38.
Even in a state of extreme weakness, such a
tantrika succeeds in this accomplishment.
Even starving, he finds his food.

39.
With his only support the recognition of the
heart, the tantrika is omniscient and in
harmony with the world.

40.
If the body/mind is ravaged by
discouragement due to ignorance, only the
completely unlimited expansion of
consciousness will dissipate a lassitude
whose source will then have disappeared.

41.
The revelation of the Self arises in the person
who is now only absolute desire. May each
of us have this experience!

42.
Then, may light, sound, form, and taste
come and impede the person who is still tied
to the ego.

43.

When the tantrika pervades everything with his absolute desire, what use are words? He has this experience on his own.

44.

May the tantrika remain present, his senses vigilantly sown in reality, and may he know stability.

45.

The person who is deprived of his power by the dark forces of limited activity becomes the plaything of the energy of sounds.

46.

Caught in the field of subtle energies and mental representations, the supreme ambrosia is dissolved, and the person forgets his innate freedom.

47.

The power of the word is always ready to veil the profound nature of the Self because no mental representation can free itself from language.

48.

The energy of the sacred tremor that passes through the vulgar person enslaves him,

whereas this same energy liberates the
person who is on the path.

49., 50.

The subtle body itself is an obstacle that is
tied to limited intelligence and to the ego.
The enslaved person has experiences that
are tied to his beliefs and to the idea that he
has of his body, and in this very way
perpetuates the tie.

51.

But when the tantrika becomes established
in the sacred tremor of reality, he liberates
the flow of manifestation and return, and in
this way takes pleasure in the universal
freedom, as a master of the wheel of
energies.

52.

I venerate the spontaneous, tremoring, and
wonderful words of my master who had me
cross the Ocean of doubt.

May this jewel of knowledge lead all beings
to reach the true nature of reality, and may
they keep this jewel in the deepest part of
their heart.[2]

The Commentary

The teaching relates to the three flows of the Spanda:

© The instructions concerning the independent existence of the Self.
© The direct perception of one's own fundamental nature.
© The universal nature reflected in the power of one's own nature.

First Flow
(Stanzas 1–16)

The Instructions Concerning the Independent Existence of the Self

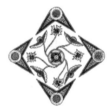

STANZA 1

The venerated Shankari (Shakti), source of energy,
opens her eyes and the universe is reabsorbed in pure
consciousness; she closes them and the universe is
manifested within her.

The Shakti is one with Shiva; the teaching is the joyous issue of their union. Whether she appears or withdraws, the Shakti escapes from the succession of time. In her breast, in the form of Kali, she does away with space-time. It is the relation of impassioned worship with the divinity or the guru that feeds our own divinity and allows us, through the mirror of this passion, to discover fundamental freedom.

The eyes open in Bhairavimudra, turned inward, without blinking, and the world is reabsorbed in pure consciousness. The eyes close, the world appears within us, for when mastery of this mudra is achieved, we are the divinity. From now on, there is no longer inner and outer, but rather, totality bathed by omnipresent consciousness. This is the secret kept by the Great Seal, the Great Cosmic Movement, the Great Configuration of the cosmos, one of the thousand names of Kali: Mahamudra. This teaching flows from the Ocean of Consciousness; it is the heart of the yoginis. Physical and mental contraction obscures perception of our innate nature and gives rise to duality. The yogin and yogini experience the nondifferentiation of states, the pure consciousness of the "I." Consciousness gleams. It cannot be said that Shankari inhales or that she exhales. The senses are the wheel of energies, the freedom of their expressions, the creativity of consciousness.

Shiva/Shakti express themselves through play and creativity in absolute consciousness. They do not have plans for the creation that emanates from them, any more than a musician has plans for the sounds that emanate from his consciousness and then from his instrument in an infinite wave. If people enter into resonance, it is because divine consciousness, the musician's consciousness, and the listener's consciousness are indivisible. The Shakti is the supreme artist; the yogini and the yogin are the supreme listeners. The Shakti is the source of the person teaching and the place of return for the sensory perceptions of the person listening. Consciousness is in total expansion when they allow their senses to vibrate in the sacred tremor, Spanda. Inner speech then ceases, the sense of the ego collapses, duality dissipates like fog in a valley when the sun suddenly appears, and silence becomes established.

The universe is uninterrupted density of consciousness fulfilled by the Self.

This first stanza contains the kernel of the teaching in its totality.

Savari sings:

> *It is neither going nor standing still,*
> *Neither static, nor dynamic,*
> *Neither substance nor nonsubstance,*
> *Neither appearance nor emptiness.*
> *The nature of all things, like space,*
> *Is without any movement.*
> *One may call it "space"*
> *But it is empty of any essence*
> *And as such it transcends definitions*
> *Such as real or unreal,*
> *Existent or nonexistent,*
> *Or anything else.*
> *Thus not the slightest distinction exists*
> *Between space, the mind, and intrinsic reality.*
> *Only their designations are different,*
> *But they are unreal and false.*[1]

One of the great intuitions of Kashmiri Tantrism was to replace linear logic with spherical, or nondual, logic. This first stanza is about the appearance and reabsorption of the universe, or the manifestation of any emotion and its withdrawal. The Tantric masters introduced the sphere into their system of thought so that things could no longer be defined in a particular manner or represent a point of spatial fixedness; each point thus remains in contact with the whole sphere in which it is navigating and ends up merging itself into the One. For a tantrika, an emotion—for example, sadness—is a prelude to joy. The idea that the world was created and that one day it will be destroyed is unfathomable because we see the creation/destruction process as a perpetual cycle. Birth and death are included in this cycle, and everything returns to absolute consciousness.

This text discusses the sacred tremor. The very characteristic of the sacred tremor is that we penetrate, thanks to it, into this spherical and nondual logic, which at first glance seems illogical because it is contrary to all that we have learned. However, the nondual view is the only way to resolve and integrate the oppositions that make us suffer so much. As soon as we penetrate into this manner of spherical thinking, we are in movement and, consequently, there is no longer any break in the fluidity of motion. There are simply moments of more or less intensity. We have the physical evidence that the body/mind is the experience. As soon as we are able to attain cyclical thinking, we can overcome the most difficult issue for a human being: that of being caught between the beginning and the end of something. What makes the practitioner suffer is that there is always a beginning of a process followed by a moment where this process reaches an end, only to be replaced by another process. According to the tantrikas, the duality that we perceive is merely a state of contraction. At the moment when the Shakti, or energy, is no longer contracted, we are able to relax, and at the same instant we experience nonduality because our body/thought is no longer limited. It is space. Our body/thought becomes spherical because we contain within ourselves all that is outside of us. We no longer perceive anything as outside of ourselves. The Tantric poets, such as Lalla, Utpaladeva, and Abhinavagupta, speak of the inclusion of the entire universe within the Self.

The whole *Spandakarika* says that the sacred tremor is the way in to this new manner of seeing and feeling things. This is not a mental process, but a dynamic that engages both the body and the mind. As soon as we experience this nonduality, even if only for a few minutes, something is unblocked. Even when contraction occurs again, the experience will stand out from everything that we have lived up to now. The idea that confusion is a contraction of the Shakti is valid for the body, the mind, and all the mind's mental creations. The Tantric texts inform us that duality is a mental fabrication, and that the body would be ready to grasp nonduality if the dictatorship of the mind did not keep us in a state of separation, in duality.

If there is such insistence on joining the body and mind, it is so that the whole person can have this experience of nonduality. Of course, when we speak of nonduality in the tantric system, we go very far, because we are not speaking of something that would be opposed to duality. If we take refuge in nonduality, as in something absolute, we are still not quite there, we still do not quite get it, because the nondual idea is to go beyond all notions. Then we will find ourselves immersed in a spherical universe and no longer in a pair of opposing concepts. We are no longer in nonduality, nor are we in duality; rather, we are now in a comprehensive experience that includes both. Once we reach this state, we realize that all oppositions are mental fabrications and that the ideas of creation/destruction, beginning/end, rise/descent, all take flight once we enter into this logic, not of mental understanding, but of direct experience.

When the Shakti opens her eyes, the universe becomes pure consciousness—which is somewhat the opposite of what one might think. When she closes them, the universe is within her. For us, it is the same thing, because the universe is in us at every moment. Once contraction ceases, we have the experience of containing everything. This is the only perception that can lead us to exhilarating serenity. The mystic stream of Mahamudra will push us toward this integration of opposites, through the most subtle strategies of the mind as well as through the yoga practices. The stanzas of the *Vijnanabhairava Tantra* are made to open this spherical space within us and to introduce us to the experience of complete relaxing that becomes the Shakti presence. When we talk about awakening, it is nothing other than this. It is to discover, in a more or less permanent manner, this comprehensiveness of the universe, which is wholly contained in our consciousness. This is not a fixed state, as we might believe, but infinite fluctuation. There is never a beginning, nor an end. If we imagine ourselves walking inside a sphere, we cannot say we left from one point and that we are going around: we can turn in all directions as if we were a gyroscope. When we enter this spherical movement, we attain something eminently alive and always moving, the essence of all things. We become caught up in this movement and, even in difficult moments, we can get a taste of what we are seeking, for what we are seeking is simply what we are. There is therefore no distance to cover; it can occur in a second. From the moment that we are completely in this spherical energy, all of life's events come to fall within it, in a new dynamic that is inexhaustible, for this new dynamic is fed from within. Consciousness is "pregnant" with the totality of the universe. Everything can arise, everything can be reabsorbed, all states become passages, crossings. And when we leave behind the perception of a fixed state, we are now necessarily in continual movement. Emotions can circulate freely, and we realize that, when we allow things to circulate, they become intimately tuned to the rapid functioning of the mind.

There are blockages and stagnation, circular repetition and routine, when we struggle against this natural rhythm of the mind. These are what cause suffering. The essential idea of Tantrism is that the things that make us suffer are blockages of the internal circular movement, blockages that we arbitrarily impose upon ourselves. This is what we call contraction of the Shakti. When there are no more blockages of internal movement, everything can circulate endlessly. We are no longer obsessed with making things fixed, and experience becomes more intense because movement can now come into all its fullness. The more we accentuate movement, the more it coincides with the true nature of the mind. This brings us that profound joy, that sensation of bliss, for suddenly everything can come forward, reveal itself, and disappear in a vast, unending movement. No longer is there localization of the body. The body becomes a much more refined instrument than it is when we are in a system of linear thought. We discover that all limits are arbitrary. We discover that there is a physical and mental expansion, absolutely limitless, into which we can enter, and which we can taste at every single moment.

STANZA 2

The sacred tremor, the very place of creation and
return, is completely limitless because its nature is
formless.

The most majestic tree is contained within a tiny seed. Similarly, the
Self, the heart revealed by the sacred tremor, possesses the capacity to
be the universal seed. All the worlds reside in the kernel of the heart.
The heart is limitless and, as it has no form, it can contain totality.

When, to us, things seem to be exterior, this is because the heart is
still deaf to limitlessness. If the world were not within us, from where
would it emerge, in what place would it be dissolved?

The sacred tremor is completely limitless because its form is so
fleeting that we cannot apprehend it. Nothing can keep the yogini and
the yogin from experiencing this on their own. Once a person becomes
peaceful, her unlimited nature emerges, and the whole cosmos recognizes her. There are no ties other than the differentiating constructions
of thought. Return to the source, and you will find the sacred tremor of
absolute freedom.

Consciousness has the nature of space. It is infinite. The body has the
nature of space, emotions and thoughts have the nature of space, sensory
perceptions have the nature of space. No one can imprison the sky using
thought; in this same way, consciousness is free of all limitation.

⚬

Virupa sang:

> But for its designation the mind is empty
> And nonconceptual, which means mahamudra.
> It is empty from the beginning, like space.
> The essence of the mind is unborn [emptiness]
> And is detached from all substantive reality.
> Like space, it is all-pervasive.
> Neither transferring nor transforming,

It has always been empty and selfless
From the beginning.[2]

The sacred tremor is something that is found on all levels, something palpable. In Tantrism, all is palpable. There are virtually no abstract notions. The idea of the masters is to introduce those who are on the path to the fact that what is being discussed in this text and in this book can be grasped by the body/mind at every moment. This is a revolutionary thought. If we seek spiritual nourishment that is purely mental, we will not find happiness or bliss, or even tranquillity. Focusing one's search on the mental aspect of the teachings brings about enormous gaps, because then nothing can be verified through the senses. The Tantric approach leads to verification in daily life, to immediate integration. Mystical movement is not intended to get us to experience extraordinary mental states of altered consciousness, but rather to plunge us into reality and to get us to discover that the absolute is found nowhere else *but* in this reality. Remember the Tantra that states, "All that is here is elsewhere. What is not here is nowhere."

From the time when the acuteness of the senses begins to open up and develop, space grows, and we realize that everything that seems mental or intellectual can be experienced physically. This is very reassuring, as we can easily get lost in such notions as "the absolute." Dozens of definitions of the absolute can be given, but when the body opens to this dimension, there are no longer any explanations to give. This is an experience that we have on our own, that we understand when we have lived it. At first, we establish all kinds of ideas for ourselves, we suppose all kinds of things. Then, one fine day, we experience it and, in the same action, the experiencer disappears. This is truly the prelude to our complete transformation.

The sacred tremor is both a prelude and an outcome. It occurs at the moment when the experience takes place. It is thus slightly odd. We have a premonition of a certain sacred tremor because something is happening in the body. Our brain, our cells, vibrate like a musical instrument, and we tell ourselves that this is the sacred tremor. Then the fact that we are in this state pushes us progressively toward something even more powerful. But the day when this really happens is yet still different. However, this whole process of setting the sacred tremor into motion is indispensable to discovering other domains that are completely unfamiliar to us. Little by little the body starts to resonate, as if all its harmonics were coming into unison in order to generate a total tremoring. When this total tremoring is born, it is as if we are introducing into our body a magic virus that is attacking all our mental constructions and relaxing them completely.

When this happens, the shock sometimes brings on intense panic, fear of the void, anxiety about something more powerful than anything we have ever known. We sense the immense power of deconstruction that the sacred tremor possesses, and this is very frightening. We sense that the system that we have forged for ourselves in order to survive is being completely upset, turned inside out, by an unknown force that is coming from the most inner part of ourselves. In these moments, a desire to retreat occurs; a wish to run away chokes us, because we feel this is irreversible. A tidal wave sweeps through our body. It is going to clean away all our established automatisms, all our fabrications. As soon as what is fabricated starts to crumble, we truly reach the state of the sacred tremor being considered in this text. Everything that is rigid in our system is volatilized.

The great trap will be the temptation to reconstruct another defense system. And to do so, we will use the teaching we have received. We will take the part that suits us, and with this part, we will reconstruct some certainty. This is the most delicate moment of the practice, because right then when we are completely open, we are overcome by the tidal wave of anxiety, and almost immediately, we reconstruct some certainty. We will do this so well that we will have the impression that our reconstruction is compatible with space.

It is, therefore, a process that unfolds in several stages. There is the first process of opening; then, an imperial need for certainty and a reoccupation of space where we can store mental objects. Soon, there will be no more room.

Then, little by little, with all our being we will understand the splendor of remaining completely outside of all systems that are built upon certainties. And when the certainties try to come back—because they always come back—we will perhaps be able to look at them with a certain irony, a certain tenderness even, noticing that they no longer work very well. Then starts the most joyous part of the practice, because we see all these conceptual pieces of old junk, with which we have worked for so long, make a desperate attempt to hang onto and then slide pathetically down the wall of the Self. There is intense happiness in participating in all these little inner catastrophes. It is also the moment of the practice when the relationship between master and disciple is most intense, because it is so delicate, so fleeting, that the connection must be very strong to avoid that space being filled again with old musty museum items. We then truly pass into another dimension, all the while seeing that what has been habitual for us until now is still occurring. Experiencing this can happen in a thousand ways. This is the flow of freedom that is starting to become established. This tremoring energy occurs, finally disallowing all new constructions.

Sacred tremor is the perfect phrase for expressing this process. Sometimes other expressions are found in the texts, like *vibration, wave, light,* and *power.* But *tremor* is easy to reach, easy to imagine. It is related to music, to love, to emotion, to the feeling of all things. The wonderful high points of our memory are the mountains of this tremoring.

When the sacred tremor occurs, we discover the ardor of the burning fire of love that is consciousness of the absolute unity of all things.

STANZA 3

Even within duality, the tantrika goes straight to the
nondual source, because pure subjectivity always
resides immersed within his own nature.

The pulsing of consciousness is the source from which the tantrika drinks; it is the manifestation of the Shakti. The worlds are not divided; all that is here is elsewhere, all that is not here is nowhere. Duality and nonduality are united within the heart of reality, like shadow and light, silence and sound, sun and moon. There is no separate reality. Everything is the expression of the supreme Shakti. Hence, the yogi and yogini never leave the fundamental intuitive sensing of the unity of all things, and it is of little importance that they are evolving in the dual universe because, in their heart, duality and nonduality are but mere concepts, empty of meaning. The whole manifestation plays within their own unlimited body, the entire cosmos navigates within the smallest particle of their body. Everything is both image and reflection, there is no place where unreality can slip in. Everything is real, both immanent and transcendent.

Our true nature is the awareness of this tremoring totality that never stops glorifying the infinite in the finite, the unlimited in the limited, the totality in the fragment. Duality thus lived ceases to limit the body and thought of the tantrika. Lack of awareness is, then, only a contraction of consciousness and of the body, but in our own nature, there is no tension, no limits at all. The great release of yoga brings us back to our absolute essence through expansion. We reach toward the infinite and we touch the heart, we come back toward our center and touch the infinite space. Nothing in reality can limit us because we see the infinite in all things.

Savari sang:
> The primordial purity of the mind
> Is the nature of space.
> There is nothing that anyone
> Can receive or reject![3]

> All the different rivers, the Ganges and the rest,
> Become one flavor in the salty ocean.

Understand that all discriminating mind, the mental events,
Become of one flavor in the expanse of intrinsic reality.[4]

For a realized mind the duality
Of meditation and meditator does not exist.
Just as space cannot perceive itself as an object,
So emptiness cannot meditate on itself.
In a state of nondual awareness
The diverse perceptions blend uninterruptedly,
Like milk and water, into the one flavor great bliss.[5]

When we take nonduality as the objective to reach, and when we desire this state, we are already lost. This stanza possesses great power to remove feelings of guilt. Previously, we had made nonduality our new ideal. Kallata, the author of the text, places us back in duality, which we had not left anyway. He releases us. There is no place that is not the Shaivite state. Spatial consciousness occupies the totality of the worlds, the totality of the senses; it includes opposites and reconciles them.

Understanding this state allows letting go of expectation, projection, and the desire to know nonduality. Once this relaxing touches the inner kernel of the person, the experience of unity can happen. In this relaxing, we will feel the freedom of passing from a momentary state of unity to a state of contraction that gives substance back to duality; then, in a successive wave, the nondual state will no doubt return. This is initiation into the releasing of physical, emotional, and mental tensions, to stop conceiving of the objective to be attained, to practice yoga and silent meditation without setting up any expectations at all, in the freedom of the moment. To let the universe glide into us without even resorting to the strategies of yoga and meditation, to arrive at pure presence. This is the entire teaching of Mahamudra.

We make too much effort; we want too much a state about which we can make a whole fantasy world. We are afraid of losing a state before we even reach it and, as soon as we do reach it, we actually do lose it. It is not we who reach the state; it is the state that reaches us. It is not we who create silence; it is silence that pervades us. Let us allow it the freedom to brush up against us, to penetrate us, to settle in within us for a few moments, to leave us, to come back. If, when silence leaves us, we have the impression that we have failed, the tension that our guilt produces prevents any return to the state of unity. This is the most difficult thing to attain: accepting the freedom of movement, the creativity of life, understanding that a fixed state, as marvelous as it might be, is not compatible with life.

Think about an Indian musician. He presents the theme of the raga; then, subtly and slowly, he explores all the expressive possibilities of the raga, he ventures out, he touches lightly, he penetrates, he withdraws, he allows himself to be taken over by ecstatic joy, returns to the most masterful variations, allows the theme to lead him to an expressive climax and, little by little, comes back down to silence. Never will he play this raga in the same way. His playing depended upon the totality of the surrounding factors—his audience, the weather, the night, the day, the scents, the sensitivity of his body, the state of relaxation of his muscles, spatiality—that were living in him on that day.

Let us enter the great spherical movement; let us forget the rectilinear pathway that assumes there is progression and the attainment of a goal. Let us be like a wave that accepts its pathway, its strength, its weakness, its freedom, the absence of choice.

Once we leave the rectilinear behind, we enter naturally into subtlety. Our meandering movement is no longer movement in a forward direction, but movement toward the living, the spontaneous, the creative. This great letting go brings us unexpected joy. It is the first sign that we accept the movement of the world, that we are leaving the domain of this ridiculous claim of wanting to control our destiny and that of others. Joy depends only upon this acceptance, only upon this movement toward fluidity, toward the spherical.

This new way of letting ourselves be will affect all the strata of our lives, which is the meaning of the Tantric approach. No areas receive special treatment. We work with the totality of what makes a human being; our yoga touches everything: beauty, violence, love, hate, giving, possession. Nothing seems out of context to us. We work with the totality of human expression. We transform nothing, we refuse nothing. We do not transmute negative emotions into their opposites. We do not have an ideal. We work with what is. Whereas at the yoga level, we work at accompanying emotions back to their return to the spatial source and thus feel that all emotions, even negative ones, lead us back to space; at the Mahamudra level, we grasp in the space of a lightning flash that emotion is spatial right from its emergence and that it remains so until its dissolution. We can no longer escape from the spacelike body: everything is inscribed therein. Everything is self-liberated at the very moment it emerges.

This is what the second stanza was telling us: when form no longer exists, there is space. What we usually try to do is introduce, at all costs, a form. But in introducing form, we automatically introduce limitation. We spend our days introducing limits. Through these limits, we introduce duality—the finished, the unfinished, the beginning, the end. We are continuously tossed about between these extremes. This state absorbs a tremendous amount of energy, exhausts us, and makes us suffer terribly.

The third stanza is also about subjectivity. In the West, we always talk about being objective, and we try to reach this ideal by learning all sorts of things. In life we make an enormous effort to be objective. In the Tantric system, on the contrary, we are told that objectivity is something compressed that is of no interest. What is interesting is pure subjectivity. We then feel destabilized because we thought the ideal was objectivity, and now we are being told that the ideal is subjectivity.

However, pure subjectivity is consciousness that is completely open. This marvelous idea means that whatever we do, we never leave this awareness. Indeed, once we reach the sacred tremor, even distraction and confusion are then imbued with consciousness. We find ourselves in space, and we return to the source being considered in this text. "Immersed in one's own nature" means that whatever the jolts or the sufferings, we cannot escape from a state of absolute calm, which is the foundation of our own nature.

It happens one day, during our practice, that we have these two experiences simultaneously. This is an extraordinary moment: we are suffering and, simultaneously, we are immersed in an ocean of tranquillity. Suffering seemed intolerable because we thought it was a state we could never bring to an end, a state dependent on others. We were waiting for others to bring an end to whatever was creating our suffering. In our case, it is completely different. We experience that it is possible to suffer, and, at the same time, to be in the state of absolute calm. Once we have lived that, even if only fleetingly, our whole relationship with suffering is transformed. Suddenly, we are much less afraid of suffering because it is no longer something that is irreversible.

As we permit ourselves to allow suffering to occur, we perceive that if we no longer constrain it in any way whatsoever, it goes away very quickly. When we become used to a certain amount of suffering, to see it—the very same suffering that we know so well, the very same suffering that can last a week—return one day and then suddenly disappear is very surprising. At the same time, the ego revolts and declares: "Well, it's my suffering after all, why is it no longer here?" We call out to it, we look for it. All of this is the experience of Tantric practice: having experiences that are completely out of the norm, outside of what we thought possible, and realizing that this is the fundamental truth of being a human.

Once we have these experiences, we get a little smile on our face when suffering returns, even if it is very violent, because we know that from now on it can leave again just as quickly as it came. We then enter into a sphere of rapid movements and acceptance. We know that this is a state that everyone goes through, but we also know that it is fleeting. And when we have had the experience several times, it brings about a sort of fundamental confidence in life, a sort of return to the Self, to one's own nature. We sense that whatever the energy entering into this sphere, it is taking part in the natural movement of being a human. Nothing is to be rejected or held onto. What makes us suffer is none other than a force that pushes us to want to choose certain things and to avoid other things, and this is precisely what obstructs the flow of energy. Indeed, as soon as a pleasant emotion, feeling, or thought comes to us, we feel the need to put it in a cage, to suspend it in our spherical space. Obviously, this does not work, and happiness escapes from us. We plunge once again into suffering. Then, as soon as we feel the two simultaneous movements, we regain our confidence. We know that, sooner or later, life will bring us something that will take us out of suffering. Sometimes even suffering runs away, because when there is the release and relaxation, it is suffering that "suffers" and finds itself in a state of contraction. One cannot suffer when the breath is calm; as soon as there is suffering, the whole body tightens up, physically as well as mentally. As soon as we experience the volatile state of suffering, it goes away. Even suffering profoundly, for very good reasons, no longer succeeds in paralyzing us. How terrible! Then we realize how much we are dependent upon this suffering, how much we feed it, how much we flatter it to make sure that it will not abandon us—because suffering makes us sure that we are still alive. And of course, feeling that we are finally, perhaps, going to stop suffering will become an anxiety in the course of our practice.

STANZA 4

All the relative notions tied to the ego rediscover their peaceful source deeply buried under all the different states.

To establish a truth, an ego is necessary. Without an ego, the truth is all truths together. When we believe that all is true, we find the peaceful source where images dissolve one after the other. The space of our thought becomes infinite, a place to pass through, a riverbed that no longer seeks to know if the leaves and the twigs are "true." Hence, in this flow, relative notions get lost in the sky of totality. Who would want to fight, who would want to win? Waking, dreaming, and profound sleep are united by the absence of contradictory truths. Everything is true, everything is illusory, everything is real. This reality encompasses the material and the immaterial, the movable and the immovable. Consciousness is the river of unity; there is no longer any division in the yogini and yogin's life.

Saraha said:

> One neither looks elsewhere for nonconceptual mind
> Nor searches for its natural qualities
> Except by clearing adverse conditions.
> This one cannot discover through the tantras and the sastras.
> A mind without craving and clinging
> Remains free from existential defilement.
> The essential nature of the mind is detached
> From either good or bad qualities.
> To actualize this, no process of inner development is
> 　necessary,
> For the mind that has abandoned such processes
> Is the great and sublime bliss.
> He who turns his mind into a nondiscriminatory state
> Will attain supreme enlightenment.[6]

Savari continued:

> Ah, does a mystic who has realized the pure nondual state
> Need to accept or reject anything?
> I have neither objectified nor abandoned any realities;
> You, my son, should not command anyone to do otherwise.[7]

And finally, Virupa said:

> Actualize significance of that which is pure, ultimate reality!
> This is the best means to let awareness
> Remain blissfully in its natural state
> Without any concern for abandoning or accepting,
> Acting or obstructing.[8]

The ego is the most erectile part of the body! Taking an entire day to observe everything that goes on there, developing immediate awareness of the spasmodic activities of the ego is a marvelous practice. Lalita Devi often asked me to describe to her in a lot of detail a slice of my life of a few hours. This could take a long time because she wanted to know absolutely everything. She wanted as precise an account as possible of all sensory, emotional, and mental activity. I would then realize how alert the ego really is, and sometimes a mere breeze was enough to make it suddenly surge up again.

This is why observing the various upsurges of the ego leads to the realization that the sacred tremor can move in and become established once the ego takes a hike, once the body finds its spatial dimension again. We all know how easy it is to provoke someone's ego, how the slightest comment is liable to make it react. The ego is like those mustard jars sold in novelty stores that a devil pops out of when we open the lid. But when we become sensitive to the spherical approach to life, this phenomenon subsides, and then stops.

Knowing that the ego becomes aroused through criticism as well as through compliments, when we start to hear things without the ego reacting, we have a strange—to say the least—experience of abandoning the body, because this sets off a relaxation of the breath. The effect is curious because we are involved in what we are hearing, but the devil does not spring out of the mustard jar. There are two joint happenings. We feel that this is intended for the ego, but we do not really know where the ego is anymore. The ego has gone for a walk. It will be back later. Maybe it went to take the dog out or to rent a video. Its energy gets lost in the gigantic sphere, like a tiny spermatozoid in infinity, seeking something and finding nothing: he loses his mind and ends up exploding.

STANZA 5

In the absolute sense, pleasure and suffering, subject
and object, are nothing other than the space of
profound consciousness.

In the unity of the uninterrupted flow of consciousness, the different
states are not divided, they are one and the same dynamic carried by the
spacelike body which contains the totality of the universes, thoughts,
emotions, and sensations. Discriminating between positive and negative
movement only dims the power of the wave that carries us unceasingly
to the finite and the infinite and reconnects them in an ecstatic harmony. The yogin and the yogini seek neither to attain illusory fixedness
nor to cut themselves off from the world of thought, emotion, or cor-
poral experience. There is only one motion, one flow, which at every
instant attests to our absolute essence.

Je Gampopa said:
> The mind has to be let loose without directing.
> Sustained mindfulness has to be cast away
> Without objectifying it.
> The mind has to be left in its ordinary state without
>   meditating.
> Thus, with nothing controlling it,
> The mind is joyous and at ease.
> Where there is no nurturing of mindfulness,
> There is no fear of distraction;
> Where there is no separation between absorption and
>   postabsorption,
> There is no intermediate state;
> Where there are diverse perceptions in the expanse of reality,
> There is no acceptance or abandonment;
> Where there is a false designation of everything,

There is an awareness of the falsity.
For the one who realizes the unreality of the mind,
All cosmic appearances and existences are an expanse of
  emptiness;
For the one who does not ascribe values to discrimination,
All [emerging thoughts] are spontaneously released;
For the one who shuns inner yearning and attachments,
All things remain harmonious evenness;
For the one who has realized all these,
Meditation is an uninterrupted stream.[9]

The fifth stanza should relieve us completely, because we might believe that being in pleasure and suffering simultaneously is something terrible. But no, Kallata eliminates this opposition. He says that to be subject and object in duality is profound consciousness. Before we even start, we have already attained the objective. It is wonderful that this objective is totally internal, that it is our source, the source of all things. Devi often told me, "The day that you stop thinking I can do something for you, that is when this will become very interesting."

This is a distinctive feature of Tantrism that the masters very much insist upon, so that we can overcome dependence, realizing little by little that the treasure we are looking for is inside us, and that all we have to do is contact it in snatches so that it will truly appear once on that great day. Over the course of your practice, you will realize this physically. You will then be comforted that you are no longer completely dependent upon he or she who suckles you and to whom you are so attached that you cannot experience the love you seek, as this love cannot be found in someone else, the so-called master, but only within yourself. Abandon the hope that someone will pour over you the fine ambrosia considered in these texts; taste it at the source of your own heart. Fundamentally, there is neither master nor disciple, although there is sometimes a non-neurotic connection between two people who walk together in space. It can be said that this is love.

The day that we realize this, we will strap on the seven-league boots because we will have become independent. The beauty of Tantrism is that the masters make every possible effort to ensure that their disciples acquire real autonomy, so that no subjugation will be established. This requires constant vigilance. We are intoxicated by dependence. The great spatial freedom, who has experienced it? Once we have this taste of freedom on our tongue, we slip into this cyclic energy and we realize that, fundamentally, no outer nourishment can fulfill us. We then experience this marvelous state toward which Devi was continually pushing me: absolute confidence in oneself, in one's incandescent kernel, free and absolute.

This is a difficult stage because we are conditioned to doubt our completeness. Harder still is to trust the idea that we have all this richness within us and that a text like the "Sacred Tremor" is only one jolt of this energy, the expression of our fundamental liberty—as if the knowledge came from our body, as if we had written this text ourselves, as if it were a manifestation of our absolute consciousness.

Kallata reintroduces us to the presence of the senses. It is true, all that is being considered here can pass only through the senses. If we deeply enter into this text, we will have the sensation that it is about our own substance, even though someone else wrote it. We understand with our whole body, with our whole mind. We feel, while reading, that this text is the image of what we deeply are. One day, confidence begins to bloom, then flowers. We then lose the idea of separation, and we get a taste of totality, space. There is no longer a connection that keeps being severed; there is, on the contrary, a process that never stops evolving over the course of a life, movement that takes us always farther toward new experiences. Gradually, things open up, and the process is never over. Never will we attain a fixed state of tranquillity or absolute happiness, because process itself *is* this absolute happiness. Once this fact is accepted, we become completely fluid, opposites subside, joy becomes stronger and stronger, and inconceivable freedom emerges.

STANZAS 6 AND 7

To grasp this fundamental truth is to see absolute
freedom everywhere. Thus, the activity of the senses
itself dwells in this fundamental freedom and pours
forth from it.

In this way, the world of the yogin and yogini is a world of fullness
where no manifestation is considered to be separate from the absolute
condition. Everything is the manifestation of the Shakti-Shiva union.
Nothing is a threat to the unlimited, because everything resides within
it, just as the divine embryo resides in our hearts. Every act, every perception, every movement of the senses is the actualization of the divine.
This activity of the senses that liberates the tantrika is not different
from the process that binds, ever more profoundly, the person who has
not yet realized her divine nature. The pleasures of the senses tied to the
ego empty the limited person's heart, and her divine energy becomes
foreign to her; whereas these pleasures endlessly fill the heart of the
yogin and yogini, whose ego, reaching toward the infinite, is nothing
other than absolute nature. The goddesses unceasingly bring back to
our heart the whole manifestation in a continual offering to the inter-
twined Bhairava and Bhairavi. The heart is ultimate consciousness, the
unequaled, the foundation of everything that exists, the Shaktichakra,
the wheel where the goddesses blossom out, unceasingly going out to
harvest the world in order to offer its essence to the divine in the temple of the heart. The heart quivers, tremors, blazes: This is the continual manifestation of the Spanda.

Everything that brings pleasure to the heart tunes the cosmic instrument of consciousness. The person whose heart overflows no longer
aspires to any kind of realization. Centered on the goddess, she allows
all that is manifested to flow within her and in this way reaches the
unlimited. This is the great expansion where the flames of the heart
carry each sensation to its incandescence, and then offer them to the
infinite space of the heart. The goddesses then go toward the world to

harvest more flowers in a never-ending motion. This is the fire of the heart.

⟨ɛ⟩

Yung Chia Hsuan Chueh sang:

> *Have you not seen the idle man of Tao who has nothing to*
> *learn and nothing to do,*
> *Who neither discards wandering thoughts nor seeks the truth?*
> *The real nature of ignorance is Buddha-nature,*
> *The illusory empty body is the Dharma body.*[10]

⟨ɛ⟩

As always, we are reintroduced to this presence of the senses. Everything under consideration here can only pass through the senses! When all the senses and the mind are completely open, we experience this inner activity, which unendingly puts us back in touch with the sacred tremor.

The sacred tremor is not something we will find and then lose. In the beginning, however, we will have an impression of having tremored with great intensity for a given moment and then losing this tremoring. But gradually we will understand that in the Tantric quest we develop the keenness of the senses and also the feeling that the absolute is right there, even at the heart of the darkest night. From then on, we start to slow down the tremoring at the very heart of the deepest shadows. All we have to do is reach out our hand for the fruit to be there and for us to be able to taste it. Thus, we progressively leave behind all the worries and anxieties that are tied to interruption; the vibrational power of the sacred tremor grows stronger and starts to flow into our whole life. To grasp this fundamental truth is to see absolute freedom everywhere.

STANZAS 8 AND 9

Therefore, the person who rediscovers this essential
sacred tremor of consciousness escapes the dim
confusion of limited desire. Liberated in this way from
the multiplicity of impulses tied to the ego, he
experiences the supreme state.

Desire, liberated from its ties to the ego, realizes that it has no other
aspiration than the fullness of Mahamudra and, as it sees in the same
impulse that this plenitude is innate and limitless, it no longer aspires to
any realization whatsoever. There is no longer anything but intimate
vibration, continuous sacred tremoring, and the absence of localization
in time and space. This is the integration of Mahamudra.

Abhinavagupta said:
> *Right from the start, situate yourself outside of spiritual*
> *progression,*
> *Outside of contemplation,*
> *Outside of seeking,*
> *Outside of skillful speech,*
> *Outside of meditation on the divinities,*
> *Outside of concentration and recitation of the texts.*
> *What is, tell me, the absolute reality*
> *That leaves no room for any doubt whatsoever?*
> *Listen carefully!*
> *Stop becoming attached to this or that,*
> *And, dwelling in your true absolute nature,*
> *Take pleasure peacefully in the reality of the world!*[11]

This text talks a lot about desire and the senses. However, it is difficult to understand how to include the activity of desire and the senses in a mystical journey. Indeed, we imagine that every outburst of desire or the senses is an obstacle to realization. This is what a great number of mystics have experienced, and suffered from, because if we slice off a part of our being on the path, the day comes when our demons destroy the work of years of austerity. Tantrikas have certainly had the experience of completely removing themselves from the world in order to avoid impulses and in order to attain something intense, something pure, something released from the body, from the senses, and from reality. But over the course of centuries, they reconsidered this issue. Thanks to their spherical logic, in which everything is included, they discovered that we can also follow a mystical path by using the senses. And not only by using them, but by going much further, much deeper, in their use.

Rather than getting rid of the issue, they went around and around with the senses and desire, until they fully grasped that the nature of desire was this incandescence, this sacred tremoring. They realized that the problem was not desire, but what they called *limited desire*. This is a magnificent advance; the so-called pernicious, dangerous desire became a fundamental energy of Tantrism by being freed from dependence upon an object. We have trouble understanding that there can be desire without there being a specific object. Of course, at the beginning of the quest, we will come into tremoring via an object. But little by little, we will be freed from the object and will come to a vibrational creativity where objects appear like dancers and disappear into the space of our sacred tremoring. By this very process, we will strengthen the sacred tremoring even more; whereas, according to the old logic, when there is desire and no object, there is suffering and there is loss, because something is missing.

The great subtlety of the Tantric masters was to take the whole of human passions and to ask themselves these questions: "How to make it so that all is used, nothing is denied, nothing is rejected? How to make it so that we will not find ourselves one day face to face with our own demons, who always come back in hordes to destroy the quest?"

The answer is truly a great finding: we penetrate the real, we touch it with our whole being, and there we discover the absolute. Before this inspired turnaround—and also after—the absolute was considered to be something far off that we desired to release from any too-human aspects in order to be certain to reach a state that was not tainted by suffering. This is the story of the invention of the gods.

The Tantric approach, on the contrary, is to engage ourselves completely with our human characteristics and to accept the whole of what we are. But instead of using this energy in a materialistic way, which brings about suffering, lack, and frustration, we try to find a way for it to reach a much more powerful level of incandescence without causing any of the usual effects related to a limited vision of things. By putting everything that makes a human being into this mystical sphere, the Tantric masters found a possible way to escape from the negation of human urges. They tried to understand all these impulses deeply so that they could act as fuel on the mystical path.

As the reader may have noticed in this text, they even provided a few warnings about the inappropriate uses of the senses and desires, uses that limit us even more and plunge us once again into profound suffering. Once we start to understand this dynamic, we realize that there really is no place for sublimation. There is simply the act of looking deeply at what is there and of allowing whatever has remained buried to come up out of the ground and open like a budding flower. In order for this opening to take place, there is only one thing we have to do: release ourselves from objectives, goals, spiritual greed, and possessiveness.

After a period of great panic in the beginning, we realize that when desire is not limited by an object, there is no reason for it to stop. Generally, when a desire is manifested toward a specific object, sooner or later the desire comes to an end. Reality arrives at this point to feed our incandescence through all aspects of life, thereby allowing all impulses in this formless and limitless sphere to manifest themselves and to evolve freely. From the yoga perspective, there are three special love partners to be favored: chaos, fear, and space. The first two will perhaps leave us one day; the third is absolutely loyal.

STANZA 10

Then the heart realizes that the true innate nature is
both the universal agent and the subjectivity that
perceives the world. Thus immersed in understanding,
it knows and acts according to its desire.

The heart realizes that there is no distance between the divine and the profane. Divine is he who perceives the world, for he perceives only the reflection of the divine within him. The tantrika is Shiva/Shakti. No duality. No separation. No creator, no created being. The great spatiality. We are simultaneously the divine, the temple, and the worshipper.

If, within this tangled ball of sensations and impulses, the results are disastrous in the everyday, it is because there is always this erectile ego that grasps onto our energy, itself ready to take off, and the ego forces that energy to take a direction affected by thought. This energy, which had been pouring forth into the sphere, finds itself being hijacked by the ego toward a specific goal. It is easy to become aware of this phenomenon within the context of any of the human desires. All one has to do is to observe how the ego becomes erect as desire manifests itself, and how, the more desire grows, the more strained the ego becomes. There is a kind of electrical dynamic because the striving of the ego is such that one cannot help but grasp at the object. Right here is the whole tragedy of desire: its tie to the ego drives us toward our own unhappiness.

When we talk about passion, we have trouble believing that passion does not equal suffering, which makes sense, given the Latin etymology of the word: *passio* comes from *pati*, which means "to suffer." We cannot quite see that passion, after its wonderful blossoming, does not have to end in pain. Tanktrikas, on the other hand, think that once passion is capable of tricking the ego—of outdoing it—then passion can lead us toward the infinite. When desire escapes the ego, there is no shrinking. We no longer have the impression that the different openings of the body are being tightened. Passion explodes all the set frameworks, everything that is dependent upon the ego.

Indeed, this is something that we can experience at any given moment in our lives: to see how passion makes us suffer, or suddenly in a moment of grace, how it allows us to free ourselves from suffering. This is a wonderful moment, a yoga moment. Once passion is freed from suffering, it becomes even more intense. Not finding an airport to touch down at, the plane called "PASSION" then flies endlessly around and around in space. There are no more forced landings; rather, there is now an impassioned energy that continually quenches our thirst. One of Kali's names is "She who knows the nature of passion." Some twenty of Kali's names are directly tied to passion, which affirms that this impassioned energy, when we succeed in attaining it, is the essential place of the quest.

Sometimes we burn our wings badly because we cannot manage to free ourselves from the ego, and so we create suffering. At that instant, it is possible to come back to the feeling of globality in order to perceive that the energy put out into space can no longer be fixed—because the sphere is limitless. The Tantric quest entails liberating all of our bursts of energy. One we have understood this through our own experience, we perceive that our impulses subsist if they have the freedom of no longer having to be directed toward a single, specific, limited place.

This is a fundamental experience in the quest, this managing of the continual effervescence—which obviously also experiences calamities and setbacks—this sacred tremoring that never stops. The kundalini, which seems too mysterious to us, is just that: sacred tremoring that soars in limitless, formless space. The tantrikas say that this spherical kundalini, which unfurls from the heart and permeates the totality of space, is quite simply absolute love. Absolute love is neurotic love—whose incandescence we are very familiar with, as well as its torments—but neurotic love whose limits have quite simply exploded and evaporated: unhealthy love thus becomes absolute love.

In the freedom of being, desire no longer has an object and necessarily attains something universal. It is propelled within this spherical energy and can pour forth infinitely without there being any fixedness. There is then a blossoming of all the cells of the body, which then, in turn, experience joy. It is not joy for one thing or another, but simply the state in which energy flows freely, a state that makes us joyous because of the circulation of desire all through the cosmic body.

Sometimes, when we think about a mystic living alone, such as Devi did, we think that it must be terrible to be all alone in her hut, in the forest, on her mountain. Or, we think that it must be idyllic. The truth is probably between the two: it depends upon the moment. In the beginning, it is extremely difficult; there is an explosion of desire, fear, anxiety, solitude. But little by little, everything is freed in space; all impulses and all inner activity find a new playmate in the game: all of reality. Shimmering leaves, water, the sky, the earth, the clouds become our partners in love, and this relationship is so intense that the flow of energy happens continually.

At times, we think it is impossible to live without physical contact. This is because we do not realize to what extent the ascetics experience unlimited exchange of love. Their whole body is engaged in this impulse, in this sacred tremoring. There is never any end, any obstacle, any stop, any frustration. Nor is there ever any accumulation of sexual energy because this energy is disseminated all day long in this loving contact with the world. This continual vibration rids the ascetics of the problem of abstinence because they have completely integrated their sexuality, by depriving it of object, direction, and form. It pours forth in a continued motion of pleasure in reality. It is present night and day. Every sound that reaches a tantrika's ears is a loving relationship, every shimmer of light, every scent, every vibration is permanently in tune with totality. All day long there is this continued sacred tremor, which makes it possible to live the most intense, ascetic, and loving life there is, in solitude.

STANZA 11

How can this wonder-filled tantrika, who always comes back to his own fundamental nature as the source of all manifestation, be subject to transmigration?

The supreme state is not found outside of oneself, but is the original and intimate nature of our being. To abandon all seeking is the only way we can relax ourselves enough that the realization of our innate nature can flower. Desire freed from its state of tension no longer goes toward things, but everything quickens within desire like a continuous offering. This is the essence of the heart of the yoginis, the teaching of the simple fact of the beauty that pours out within us like a continuous ambrosia. The tantrika receives beauty like the earth receives the moon, the sun, and the rain, in the continuous sacred tremor of vibrating and living matter. There is nothing inanimate. All is radiating sacred tremoring— people, mountains, rivers, and emotions. The clouds and the body are atoms bound by wonder, like the sky uniting the stars.

Tao-sin said:
> The body and the mind, in their slightest movements,
> Are forever found at the place of awakening.
> Our behavior itself is the awakening:
> There is no other Buddha than the heart.
> All phenomena are nothing but the heart.
> Dwell in this state of consciousness,
> And all the knots of passion will untie themselves naturally.
> In a grain of dust

All the worlds can be found,
And all the universes are contained in the tip of one of your
    hairs.
There is no obstruction.
Do not evoke the Buddha,
Do not grasp at the mind,
No mental strategies,
Nor reflections,
Nor meditative practice,
Even less, distraction.
Abandon yourself to the flow of things,
Without restraining the thoughts!
Everything is pure!
The natural and immaculate clarity of the mind emerges![12]

The state in which a given tantrika finds himself, even within society, is exactly this state of joy, of marveling, of jubilation. All his experience is like a spring that is continually regenerating itself and encouraging him to come to know the limitless in the most banal experiences. Often we imagine that the mystic life involves intense moments of encounters with the divine. For tantrikas, the mystic life is drinking a glass of water, putting one's feet in the river, sitting at the foot of a tree or on the terrace of a café, listening to the night, waiting for the bus, looking at the stars, walking, eating. Becoming an ordinary person again.

Within the framework of society, it means living very normally. Tantric masters keep working, at the same time teaching a few disciples. Sometimes they have very simple jobs, because they are people from all walks of life: garbage men, butchers, civil servants, prostitutes, engineers. They find fulfillment in making sandals, cooking *galettes,* spinning pots, or selling lentils. It is thus truly possible to live this fulfillment in the most everyday reality.

The ideal of the tantrika is to find the absolute, right there within the everyday—not to wait for fleeting revelations and so-called altered states of consciousness. Wonder occurs when we succeed in tasting the nectar of the loving relationship that we develop with each thing or person or object that is before us at this very moment. This is what changes life completely, because otherwise we are always in search of something more. And when we obtain it, we are still unsatisfied. We then seek something even more spectacular, and this is how we end up being continually unhappy.

This does not mean, of course, that we must be satisfied with something that absolutely does not suit us. We must not confuse lifeless resignation with this ideal. If we can communicate completely with all the ordinary aspects of life, we are great mystics. The details then become much less important, as wonder, constant joy, and the sacred tremor are maintained by continued contact with the everyday, which ceases to be ordinary at the moment we really taste it.

Stanza 11 considers the subject of transmigration—which occurs occasionally in the Tantric texts—and asks clearly: "How can a wonder-filled tantrika be subject to transmigration?" Does this mean that those who are not wonder-filled are subject to transmigration? No, this is a Tantric mystery. At times it is said that there is transmigration; other times it is said that the idea of transmigration is a "hitching post for asses" (Abhinavagupta). Do not count on me to tell you!

STANZAS 12 AND 13

If the void could be an object of contemplation, where
would the consciousness that perceives it be?
Therefore, consider contemplation of the vacuity as an
artifice of a nature analogous to that of a profound
absence from the world.

The void is a cold, hard space; spatiality, a vibrant, living space. There is no difference between the void and spatiality. Space contains the worlds, beauty, violence, and fear, wonderment, love, and passion. All these impulses are the continuous sacred tremor. The person who is attached to an objectless void hardens her heart; the person who perceives a void that includes all of manifestation recognizes the divine in herself. To leave behind all oppositions is to recognize that samadhi is the only reality, since the source of all reality is found there. Going in this way toward the source of all things, the yogi and the yogini are no longer in opposition to the world: the universe lies in each of their cells like an embryo in the womb of the Goddess. The body is but a bringing together of goddesses and gods. There is neither birth nor death.

Niu-tou sang:

> *No need to seize the mind*
> *Nor to restrain it to become peaceful,*
> *Then peacefulness comes!*
> *To be mindless,*
> *Is to be void of object.*
> *Being void of object is virgin nature,*
> *Virgin nature is the Great Way!*
> *The nature of the absolute,*
> *Is spontaneity!*
> *There is no place*
> *That is not the Way!*
> *When your palm is turned toward the sky,*
> *No one asks you where it has gone!*
> *The nonestablishing of a vehicle,*
> *Is what I call the supreme vehicle!*
> *Fire ravages the mountains,*
> *Wind snaps the trees,*
> *Avalanches bury the wild beasts,*
> *Floods drown the reptiles.*
> *With such a mind, one can kill.*
> *But if the least hesitation remains,*
> *If the idea of life and death exists,*

Then an acting mind exists,
And killing an ant in these conditions is a crime.
The bee gathers nectar from the flowers,
The birds feed on sweet chestnuts,
The buffalo on beans,
The horse on prairie grasses.
Without the idea of possession,
A mountain belongs to you.
Without this freedom, a leaf ties/binds you!
The sky encircles the earth,
Yang is joined to Yin,
Rain flows in the gutters,
Springs pour into the streams.
When passions bring about differentiation,
Even the union with your own wife soils you.
If you cling to the existence of the mind,
The latter/It will exist even in samadhi.
If you free yourself from the mind,
Even in reflection, you will be free!
The wind has no mind.
The master allows his thoughts to appear.
If, at the moment of death,
You hold back sorrows,
You will give rise to the ego.
If you understand these things,
Movement and immobility will be in tune with the Way.
There is neither obstacle nor obstruction!
Therefore, eliminate your own views
Rather than reflecting upon the views of others![13]

These stanzas of the *Spandakarika* are a shaft aimed against the Buddhists who, between the eighth and twelfth centuries, were extremely powerful in Kashmir. There was a certain rivalry between them and the

Tantric masters, even if, elsewhere, some Tantric masters became the disciples of Buddhist masters. Abhinavagupta, for example, had among his numerous masters a Buddhist master. The Sufis were also very powerful in Kashmir, but the Tantric masters got along better with them in terms of their ideas and their practice of sacred dance. Be that as it may, between the nonself—the Buddhists' vacuity—and the Self—the tantrikas' reality—there was friction. Certainly absurd!

Some Buddhist masters were more open than others, and the greatest declared that the nonself was a trapdoor, a dark cavern. To understand the void with nonconsciousness seemed, in any case, excessive to the tantrikas. This is why they introduced consciousness, reality, and the Self: three very palpable elements. One of the names of Shiva is, nevertheless, the "Great Void." Was Shiva a Buddhist? The tantrikas made the void something inhabited because they talk about it as space, as do the Ch'an masters. When spatiality is under consideration in the *Vijnanabhairava Tantra*, it is a void containing the whole universe, and this void is consciousness, the Self. The Self contains the void, the nonself, plenitude, the worlds, the Buddhists, the Sufis, the Christians, the Jews, and the tantrikas! The mystical experience is one; abolishing all dogmatic limitations, it is silent fusion, the annihilation of all disputing.

Tantrikas are not much in favor of the idea that one must be seated in meditation in order to enter vacuity. Like many of the Ch'an masters, they sometimes make fun of sitting and say to anyone who will listen that a few decades of sitting are useful. Sometimes they are against meditation and say that it is useless to meditate before the awakening. One may wonder what purpose would it serve after? And yet, they have said this! They are incessant provokers! When Kallata speaks of a nature analogous to that of a profound absence from the world, this means, in certain translations at least, a state analogous to deep sleep. However, it is not exactly that because, for tantrikas, absolute consciousness exists even in deep sleep. It is more like an absence from the world in the waking state. Which is even more powerful because one is supposedly here, but one is nowhere. Therefore, meditate seriously! Sitting is wonderful, indispensable, and completely useless. Understand the matter for yourself.

STANZAS 14, 15, AND 16

Actor and action are united, but when action is dissolved by abandoning the fruits of the act, the very dynamic that is tied to the ego exhausts itself, and the tantrika who is absorbed in this profound contemplation discovers the divine tremor liberated from its ties to the ego. The profound nature of action is thus revealed, and he who has interiorized the movement of desire no longer knows dissolution. He cannot cease to exist because he has returned to the profound source.

Thus, in this great unity, everything touches everything else. A world, a movement of the body, where emotions pour out from the infinite, navigate through the infinite, end in the infinite, only to give rise to another movement. Act and actor, subject and object, perception and perceiver are united. This is the realization of Mahamudra. All actions are like a feather floating at the will of the breeze in a parade of mountains. They never cease crossing the sky. At the profound source, everything rediscovers the nature of space.

Mahasitha Shang specified that aspirants on this path should behave as follows:

To behave as a wounded deer.
A wounded deer shuns companions and shows no interest in anything else. Thus a meditator should live by himself, not depending on

friends, and should abandon any material aims for this life, aims that would help vanquish his enemies, protect his friends, and flatter his benefactors.

To behave like a lion.
A lion is not afraid of any other animals such as deer or wild beasts. Thus a meditator should fear neither external obstacles [to his performance] created by human or nonhuman beings, nor internal obstacles arising from his own deluded discrimination.

To behave like the wind blowing through space.
The wind blows freely through the expanse of space. Thus the meditator should let his thoughts flow freely and openly without any attachment to his body, possessions, happiness, or fame.

To behave like space.
Space is without any support. Thus the meditator should neither direct his mental focus toward any specific object nor create a mental support for any image such as a visualized form or a formless object. Neither should he direct his mental focus toward any specific action.

To behave like a crazy person.
A mad person lacks any objective direction. Thus a meditator should not have any attachment to anything, such as affirmation or rejection, acceptance or abandonment.

These five principles are considered to be a means of sublimating any emerging perceptions and emotions arising from adverse external or internal conditions, thereby greatly enhancing one's vision of abiding reality.[14]

Not only the Buddhists, but also the tantrikas and the Taoists, talk a lot about nonaction. This is a concept that is misunderstood if we think that it means no action at all. Nonaction does not mean striving for a sort of passivity, and trying not to act. On the contrary, it is about throwing oneself into action and forgetting completely why one is taking that action and what one wants to obtain by it. That is, it means freeing oneself from the fruits of the action. It is a little like the object of desire from which we free ourselves by experiencing energy without a goal. At that moment, say the masters—and we can verify this on our own—we experience the grace of movement. Indeed, a movement that is determined by a goal is disharmonious, whereas a completely gratuitous action reaches a different space, a grace that is impossible to find when we are constrained by the presence of the object to be obtained. What is meant here is to enter into the action, liberate the objective, and find the grace, the beauty, of the everyday gesture. Then, suddenly, there is contemplation because there is this grace. And once there is contemplation, there is the sacred tremor. It all goes together. If we try to feel the sacred tremor without considering its relationship to action, we will at times have vague sensations of sacred tremoring, but we will not find this fundamental sacred tremoring that we can maintain entirely throughout the everyday.

Reaching an occasional state of peace in meditation is a good start, but what is wonderful is to live it within daily activities. It is important that the sacred tremor not be a quasi-miraculous state, which we attain during a moment of grace, but that it become almost ordinary, perceived at the occurrence of any contact with things and beings. Then we can say that we are in meditation, because all of reality is transformed. Our presence in the world becomes so open, intense, and refined that the sacred tremoring is continual.

Mind, Empty Like Space

The great yogini Machig Labdrön lived in the second half of the eleventh century in the province of Lab, in Tibet. She is one of the essential links in the transmission of Mahamudra. Her song reveals its secrets with a sparkling liveliness. This text is the last teaching she gave at the age of ninety-nine, before disappearing into space.

Fortunate sons, keep this in your heart.
My instructions in Chöd,
Are the authentic teachings of Mahamudra [phyag rgya chen po].
This Mahamudra cannot be explained in words.
It cannot be explained, but it is like this:

> Phyag *is the nature of emptiness* [of the mind].
> Gya *is liberation from the vastness of samsaric* [appearances].
> Chen po *is the inseparable union* [of appearances and emptiness].
> *Primordially co-emergent,* [this inseparability] *like empty space*
> *Does nothing, is not dependent on anything.*
> *In the same way, mind itself,* [natural and co-emerging]
> *Has no support, has no object;*
> *Let it rest in its natural expanse without any fabrication.*

When the bonds [of negative thoughts] *are released,*
You will be free, there is no doubt.

As when gazing into space,
All other visual objects disappear,
So it is for mind itself.
When mind is looking at mind,
All discursive thoughts cease
And enlightenment is attained.

As in the sky all clouds
Disappear into sky itself:

> *Wherever they go, they go nowhere,*
> *Wherever they are, they are nowhere.*

This is the same for thoughts in the mind:
When mind looks at mind,
The waves of conceptual thought disappear.

As empty space
Is devoid of form, color or image,
So too, mind itself
Is free of form, color or image.

As the heart of the sun
Cannot be veiled by an eternity of darkness
So too, the realization of the ultimate nature of the mind
Cannot be veiled by an eternity of samsara.

Even though empty space
May be named or conventionally defined,
It is impossible to point it out as "this."
It is the same for the clarity of mind itself:
       Although its characteristics may be expressed,
It cannot be pointed out as "this."

The defining characteristic of mind
Is to be primordially empty like space;
The realization of the nature of the mind
Includes all phenomena without exception.

Once discursive thoughts are totally abandoned,
Dharmakaya is no other than that.
Once the five poisons are totally abandoned,
The five wisdoms are no other than that.

Once the three poisons are totally abandoned,
The three kayas are no other than that.
Once conventional mind is totally abandoned,
Buddhahood is no other than that.

Once samsara is totally abandoned,
Nirvana is no other than that.
Once mental agitation is totally abandoned,
Skillful means are no other than that.

Once emptiness is totally abandoned,
Discriminating wisdom [prajna] is no other than that.

Once mind is totally abandoned.
Fearsome places are no other than that.

Once virtue and nonvirtue are totally abandoned,
Gods and demons are no other than that.
Once the six consciousnesses are totally abandoned,
The six classes of beings are no other than that.
Once the eight consciousnesses are totally abandoned,
The eight armies of demons are no other than that.

Once wandering thoughts are totally abandoned,
Magical displays are no other than that,
Meditative absorption is no other than that,
The practice of the four daily sessions is no other than that.

Once discursive thoughts are totally abandoned,
The practice of Chöd is no other than that.
Once mindfulness is achieved,
The level of final accomplishment is no other than that.
Once the [ultimate nature] of mind is realized,
The definitive sign of realization is no other than that.

Abandoning all bodily activities,
Remain like a bunch of straw cut loose.
Abandoning all verbal expressions of speech,
Remain like a lute with its strings cut through.

Abandoning all mental activity,
That is Mahamudra.

In the Dharma tradition of this old lady,
There is nothing other than this.

Ah, fortunate sons and disciples gathered here,
This body of ours is impermanent like a feather on a high
   mountain pass,
This mind of ours is empty and clear like the depth of space.
Relax in that natural state, free of fabrication.
When mind is without any support, that is Mahamudra.
Becoming familiar with this, blend your mind with it—
That is Buddhahood.

You may recite mantras, be diligent in offering tormas,
Be versed in the entire Tripitaka teachings,
Including the Vinaya and the philosophical schools with their
   respective tenets,
But it will not make you realize Mahamudra, the nature of
   the mind.

Attached to your own point of view,
You merely obscure the clear light of your mind.
Protecting vows which are merely conceptual
Harms samaya in the ultimate sense.
Remain free of mental fabrications, free of consideration for
   yourself.
Like the waves in the water, naturally arising, naturally
   subsiding,
Without conceptualizations, without abiding in extreme
   [views].
In the primordial purity of mind,
There is no transgression of your samaya.

Free of desire and attachment of extreme [views],
Like a single light dispelling the darkness,
You realize at once the teachings of Sutra, Tantra and all
    other scriptures.

If you aspire to this path, you will be free from the infinity of
    samsara.
If you enter this path, you will defeat all mental afflictions
    without exception.
If you achieve this path, you will attain the highest
    enlightenment. . . .

If you imagine you will practice Dharma when you have the
    leisure,
You will lose this opportunity.
Human life is wasted in the thought, "I will practice later."
What would happen if you were to die in an accident?
If you don't meditate with perseverance now,
And if you died tomorrow, who would then provide you with
    authentic Dharma?

If you don't do it yourself,
What good will the Dharma practice of others do you?
It is like a beggar's dream,
In which he is rich in splendor, food and wealth.
Upon awakening all is gone without a trace,
Like the passing of a bird in the sky.
All composite phenomena in the world are just like that.

Right now you have the opportunity.
Look for the essence of mind—this is meaningful.
When you look at mind, there is nothing to be seen.
In this very not seeing, you see the definitive meaning.

Supreme view is beyond all duality of subject and object.
Supreme meditation is without distraction.
Supreme activity is action without effort.
Supreme fruition is without hope and fear.

Supreme view is free from reference point.
Supreme meditation is beyond conceptual mind.
Supreme activity is practice without doing.
Supreme fruition is beyond all extremes.

If you realize this, enlightenment is attained.
If you enter this path [of Mahamudra], you will reach the
*   essential nature.*
You cut wrong conceptions about inner, outer and in between,
You understand all the teachings of the higher and lower paths,
You defeat the eighty-four thousand klesas,
You perfect simultaneously the symptoms,
The sign [of realization] and the level of final accomplishment
And you cross over the ocean of samsara.

This old lady has no instructions more profound than this to
*   give you.*

[Later in time:]
My authentic teaching, the unique doctrine of the unborn,
Is the greatest of all systems of profound instructions,
This separation of body and mind and its blessing
Is the greatest of all transferences of consciousness.
This offering of the bodily aggregates
Is the greatest of banquets.
This wandering in mountain solitude and fearsome places
Is the greatest of all monasteries.
This entourage of illusory gods and demons
Is the greatest of all benefactors.

This practice free of the extremes of hope and fear
Is the greatest of all virtuous activities.
This action, the unobstructed experience of single taste,
Is the greatest of all paths of action.
This essence of ultimate meaning, beyond thought and
*   expression,*
Is the greatest of all Dharma practices.

I, Labdrön, the Shining Light of Lab,
Am the greatest of all women.
Now my death in the unborn expanse
Is the greatest of all ways to pass away.[15]

Second Flow
(Stanzas 17–27)

The Direct Perception of One's Own Fundamental Nature

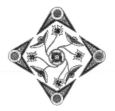

STANZA 17

The awakened tantrika realizes this continuous sacred
tremor throughout the three states.

Everything Is consciousness.

Yuanwu said:

> *The Ultimate Path is simple and easy—it is just a matter*
> *simply of whether you abandon things or pursue them.*
> *Those who would experience the Path should think deeply*
> *on this.*[1]

The three states that stanza 17 speaks of are waking, dreaming, and deep sleep. It is very often said that deep sleep is a state of nonconsciousness. But long before any research was done on dreams and sleep, the tantrikas always said that once sacred tremor occurs, consciousness pervades deep sleep as well. There is no more interruption, and the continued stream of consciousness pervades absolutely everything that we live. The sacred tremoring does not cease, even for a single moment. The power of the Shakti subsists through the three states and continually infuses the feeling of being alive.

Dreams are very important in the Tantric quest, as they are the prelude to the teachings that one receives directly in the form of dreams. It is a surprising moment in the relationship with our master when suddenly we begin not only to dream about him, but to receive his teachings in dreams. Dreams are the love chamber of the master and disciple. This sudden incandescence of dreams always comes when practice is intense. We even have the impression that we are dreaming the whole night through. Upon waking, we are tired, because an evacuation has taken place during these dreams, allowing buried issues to emerge.

When the playing field starts to level somewhat, milder, more peaceful dreams come. In these dreams, the presence of the master is so strong that one no longer suffers from distance or separation. It can be said at this time that the fruit of the relationship is ripe because a permanent joy is established, as well as total identity between master and disciple, united in the same knowledge, the same experience, the same love—and the same body, the incarnation of Shiva/Shakti, as happens in the Tantras when they separate from each other to give birth to the text, then return to the loving union. When one feels this, one no longer has the impression of possessing a separate body. A true disciple contains his master. This is something wonderful, limitless; to contain one's master is to contain the worlds. Presence lives within us, and we awake in tremoring joy, even if the memory of the dream has slipped away. This joy simply appears, flowing from this presence in the dream, which we have perhaps forgotten. When there is this feeling of lightness, waking is very subtle. We feel like we are floating.

STANZA 18

Shiva is then in loving union with Shakti in the form of
knowledge and its object, whereas everywhere else he
is manifested as pure consciousness.

In this union, the tantrika slips from one state into another without there being any break in consciousness. The awareness of consciousness is recovered in an uninterrupted stream. The states of waking, dreaming, and deep sleep are the expressions of continued consciousness. Dreams can occur just as well during the waking state as in deep sleep since consciousness envelops all that is manifested. Even in duality, nothing exists other than the expression of consciousness. There is no difference between love and pure consciousness.

The Ch'an master Dahui said:

> You don't need paraphernalia, practices, or realizations to attain it—what you need to do is to clean the influences of the psychological afflictions connected with the external world that have been accumulating in your psyche since beginningless time.
>
> Make your mind as wide open as cosmic space; detach from graspings in conceptual conscience, and false ideas and imaginings will also be like empty space. Then this effortless subtle mind will naturally be unimpeded wherever it turns.[2]

This stanza holds an allusion to the great practice of the heart, where union is permanently realized through perception of sensory objects that are brought back toward the source of the heart. It is one of the rare "secret" practices of Kashmiri yoga, a very sophisticated yoga that can only be received through direct transmission. In fact, it is so difficult to realize that, for now, the details of it are not of interest.

STANZA 19

The whole palette of the different kinds of sacred
tremoring finds its source in the universal sacred tremor
of consciousness, and in this way reaches the person.
How could such a sacred tremoring limit the tantrika?

To realize Spanda is to absorb the unlimited completely. Then all sounds are united in silence, all colors in the nature of space, all the masses of matter in the infinite fluidity.

Abhinavagupta said:

*The power that resides in the Heart of Consciousness is
freedom. This Heart is called the resting place of the
immaculate light, and pure Consciousness is not different
from all the parts of the body.*[3]

The sound palette shows very well the idea of the vibration of strings, of skin stretched over a resonance chamber. Indeed, tantrikas are similar to musical instruments. Once they start resonating, whether they are "played" by their master or by life, reality, confusion, suffering, chaos, or space, something produces unending music. At this point, they realize that the sacred tremor is not merely a kind of vibration, a repetitive sensation; on the contrary, it is a limitless feeling with a range so rich that they can have all sorts of different experiences. The tantrikas taste a tremor that is barely perceptible, an inexhaustible gamut of possibilities, like the infinity of sounds that one can bring out of a real instrument. The tantrikas feel all this.

In the beginning, the tantrika perceives only one type of tremor, a palpitation somewhere in her body, and she says to herself, "The sacred tremor feels like this." Then she feels something else and tells herself, "This is not the sacred tremor," since she believes she already knows what the sacred tremor feels like. Finally, she feels yet another type of tremor and wonders at this point if everything that she has experienced has not been the expression of the sacred tremor. In general, it is the master who gets her to see that all these experiences are connected and of the same nature, that is, completely illusory—as long as we make assets of them.

STANZA 20

And yet, this sacred tremoring itself causes people who
are subject to limited views to become lost because,
their intuition being dissociated from the profound
source, they throw themselves into the whirlwind of
transmigration.

If a person who has views that are limited by the ego attempts to actualize this teaching, he will see that in discontinuity there is transmigration. He jumps from one space to another, from one point in time to another; the flow is not continuous, and the masses of water, now forming lakes, cannot flow toward the great unity. Awareness of this momentary transmigration is the consciousness that feeds the division of a life into multiple fragments; therefore, the concept of birth and death corroborates this experience.

Utpaladeva sang:

> Who else is to be counted*
> By those resting comfortably in the celestial bliss
> Of the cool, pure, tranquil, sweet
> Sea of the nectar of devotion?

> . . . How wonderful it is that the mind, O Lord,
> In essence the seed of all suffering,
> When doused with the nectar of devotion
> Bears the magnificent fruit of beatitude.[4]

The "whirlwind of transmigration" . . . Does transmigration exist? Is it the act of the passing from one instant to the next where we are new? Is it the act of passing from one life to another? To a disciple's question about transmigration, a master replied: "Ask a master who has died. He is the only one who will be able answer you."

STANZA 21

The person who with fieriness tends toward the profound sacred tremor reaches his true nature even within activity.

Our yoga is not a yoga that is separated from the world. It is actualized in action. Meditation is a state, not an activity. For the person who enters the nonmeditation of Mahamudra, all is meditation, and action is as peaceful as sitting in solitude. At the heart of the great effervescence of the world, the person who has reached silence goes through life without the least trouble.

---

*Note from cited text: In this state, all that exists has merged into one; there is no entity separate from this.

The Ch'an master Foyan said:

There is nothing in my experience that is not true. If there were anything at all untrue, how could I presume to guide others? When I affirm my truth, there is no affirming mind and no affirmed objects; that is why I dare tell people.[5]

For those who have attained the Way, there is nothing that is not the Way. You must wait for complete nakedness before attaining realization. If you want to be in harmony with a master, simply know your own mind![6]

You should observe your present state—what is the reason for it? Why do you become confused?[7]

This is the most direct approach! Be free from both confusion and enlightenment.[8]

Someone asked Yunmen: "What is the Self of the believer?" Yunmen replied: "The mountains and the rivers, the whole Earth."[9]

Stop all seeking. It is a sickness. Then monkey mind will stop. When you see things in this way, you will be free and independent.[10]

In this stanza, Kallata recognizes that, yes, it is easier, simpler, to experience the sacred tremor outside of activity, but that a tantrika has this experience even at the very heart of activity. Kallata abolishes the separation between the contemplative state, on the one hand, during which we have powerful sensations because we are in touch with the body, and, on the other hand, life, where we are instead in touch with what is around us. The secret is to succeed at being in activity while *at the same time* maintaining deep awareness of the body, without losing that consciousness the moment stimulation arrives. In general, this is what happens: we have this presence to inner feeling, then we come to a situation where there is a great variety of stimulations, and we get lost in order to taste what is outside.

When we enter the world with a reinforced meditative capacity, the opposite happens. Perception of everything inside is intensified, and we suddenly perceive that there is something in the universe. We enter this universe feeling intensely in touch with ourselves, even though we are perceiving what is outside. When this perception becomes very intense, the inner perception of the sacred tremor seems to grow, to the point where the sacred tremor contains everything that is exterior. Inner and outer no longer exist. Consciousness passes by objects and stimulations, envelops them completely; the sensation is extremely profound as the totality of the experience is constant presence. The perception of awareness, the sacred tremor, and all the outer stimulations are then manifested within us. No longer is there a difference between perceiver and perceived. It becomes the same consciousness. This is why the Tantric texts say that consciousness is everywhere. Nothing is found outside of oneself anymore. This is one of the secrets of the *Spandakarika*.

STANZA 22

The profound and stable sacred tremor can be reached
in extreme states: anger, intense joy, mental wandering,
or the drive toward survival.

These states are vast moments of unity. The tantrika welcomes them without losing awareness of the source, and all the manifestations autoliberate themselves in the Mahamudra. Certain disciples choose to ignore the danger by renouncing the powerful states and the larger emotions; others transform the disturbances by focusing on the divine. The tantrika takes all things as the manifestation of the infinite and, in this way, sees all emergences right from the start as the sacred path of illumination, as the expression of the limitless. It is no longer even necessary to wait for the disturbances to return to the source in order to be liberated: they are, in essence, liberation.

Saraha sang:

> *Having seen [and experienced] the bliss supreme in the act of*
> *copulation*
> *In this very place, so richly adorned by sacred gatherings*
> *(tshogs-kyi 'khor-lo),*
> *With the yogis [and yoginis] responding to each other's use of*
> *symbols, and having observed their commitment [to*
> *appreciation],*
> *He will well [understand the] coequality of worldliness and*
> *quiescence—Mahamudra.*
>
> *A [Saivite] yogi in whom a [pseudoexistential] pristine*
> *awareness [allegedly imparted to him by Siva himself] has*
> *come about, [and hence] in whom there is no fear,*
> *Will, whilst wearing the insignia of Siva [as a charm], look for*
> *a woman born in the outskirts. . . .*
>
> *Taking in her qualities he will [reciprocate by] offering his*
> *pristine awareness, Reverberating within the intensity of*
> *immediate experience, and,*
> *For the time being, he will take this pristine awareness—*
> *heightened in its sensibility through Being's genuineness*
> *[operating in it], approximating in flavor*
> *[Being's nothingness replete with everything in highest*
> *perfection]—as the Mahamudra experience.[11]*

Many of us think that to experience the sacred tremor, one must be in a state of equilibrium, presence, calm; and we imagine that intense energy, like anger or a big burst of passion, are antinomical to the Way. In Tantrism, on the contrary, the yogins entered into these states while asking what was their relationship to the Way. They found that, exactly during the fear or worry, there is a precise moment when the whole person is unified and the side issues disappear. During a state of great anger, distraction suddenly ceases to exist. Only the anger is there. The whole person is one, and he experiences the sacred tremor very profoundly. This moment, which does not last long, precedes action. As soon as the anger ends in action, he loses the united core. This is a specific moment, very fleeting, which does not extend to the whole length of the anger but, rather, prepares the person to do something. When the act of violence takes place, he has already entered chaos.

When we have the chance to become angry or afraid, we feel a gathering of energy followed by a dispersal. It is in this gathering that we can reach the sacred tremor considered in this text. This requires great awareness, because generally, awareness of the state is delayed. Once the cataclysm occurs, the energy falls off again and we say to ourselves, "I was angry!" It is only rarely that we achieve a clear awareness of our emotion in the present moment. If this were always the case, there would be no drive to action, no manifestation of the emotion outside ourselves. Anger, fear, hate, and jealousy are great gifts. Finally, we leave spiritual mirage behind. We are no longer this sanitized being smelling sweetly of lotus flower perfume. We smell like hate. We stink of it. This is reality. This is unity, at last! Transforming hate into love and compassion is like putting saran wrap over a container of rotting food; it does not resolve anything. We must go to the raw and direct feeling. There is nothing to transform. To transform is to lose the chance that we have been given to look at reality. The solution is in the problem and not in its negation. The problem is a marvelous gift.

STANZAS 23 AND 24

When the tantrika gives himself over to Shiva/Shakti,
the sun and the moon come up in the central channel.

When freedom expresses itself through everything that emerges, the
yogi and the yogini allow themselves to be carried by the dynamic of
the totality. Everything is accomplished by this absence of choice; light
and infinite, they give themselves over completely to Shiva/Shakti
because they have recognized that they *are* Shiva/Shakti. In this abandonment of all personal dynamic, the infinite emerges. The central
canal is the whole cosmos and is found both in the infinite body and in
the physical body.

Chen-houei:
> *All activity deliberated by the mind is activity of limited
> consciousness. How would that make it possible to see in
> our own nature?*[12]

In Tantric iconography, the sun and the moon symbolize the breath. The
central channel is the inner canal in which the kundalini rises. It is
through the breath that the whole process of yoga begins working. The
sun and the moon are simply the breath and the stopping of the breath.
These two sequences eventually become just one, and suddenly the person is unified and can feel the central canal intensely. Through spatiality
and freedom, this canal and the chakras begin working; but the originality of the Pratyabhijna and Spanda streams is to let the subtle energy happen rather than to force it or condition it by a specific yoga. All the
practices of Matsyendranath and the *Vijnanabhairava Tantra* will, in the
end, have the effect, through their diversity and their harmony, of sensi-
tizing the subtle body. But there is no romanticism about activating, no

directed effort for stimulating or opening. Abhinavagupta even said that pranayama was dangerous and not useful. This approach is very close to Ch'an, which avoids all the obsessions and the dreams of power developed by practices that are designed to gain us access to *siddhi*. Everything emerges spontaneously when spatial letting go occurs.

At the beginning of our time together, Devi surprised me by saying that I did not have any chakras. She cut short all illusions by incessantly bringing back the practice of the path to consciousness of all that was blocking the harmonious and spontaneous flow of being. She left no way to hide behind a practice that aims to master the world. For her, only abandonment was of interest. Of course, Matsyendranath offers a wonderful teaching on the eight chakras and the secret chakra, but all is manifested in the occurrence of spontaneity, silence, the absence of fear. Only the integration of space at the emotional, physical, and cognitive levels can open us to this teaching. The subtle body is a refined sensing of the gross body; it is not another body. There is a very small difference: this subtle gross body includes the universe.

Forget the chakras. Perception of them is completely conditioned and illusory. It depends upon your beliefs. If you believe there are seven of them, you will feel seven. If you believe there are twelve of them, you will feel twelve. If you do not believe chakras exist, you will feel a thousand chakras. What is important is that awareness become more intense, that the capacity to concentrate become keener, and this leads to the possibility of feeling intensely the openings as well as the closings. But one can have a breathing practice only when it has become something natural, as doing exercises does not necessarily bring about a true letting go of the breath. The Tantric idea is to never make anything up and to participate in the opening through presence. One cannot make up "good" breathing, pranayama or not. We enter ourselves, we descend with presence, and there we begin to feel that there are areas predisposed to vibration, to the sacred tremor.

It is as if we are an instrument without strings and we are going to buy the strings. The instrument suddenly finds its purpose because the strings are there. And the strings are the awareness that we have of the instrument. All we need to do, then, is to have this profound consciousness of the instrument, and the strings will be born of themselves. Reading the *Vijnanabhairava Tantra* makes us recognize something that was already there. This is the profound practice: a consciousness that is headed toward a state of freedom prior to all dreams of freedom and all fetishism during practice. And to give oneself over to Shiva/Shakti is to allow oneself to go toward this perception. To flow toward one's own source.

STANZA 25

At that moment, when in the sky the sun and the moon disappear, the awakened person remains lucid, whereas the ordinary person sinks into unconsciousness.

When consciousness reveals itself to the unconscious person whose actions are automatic and whose distraction from the source is permanent, there no longer exists a division between the states. The sun and the moon suddenly appear in the space of the infinite body of the yogi and the yogini.

Lalla sang:
> *The Way of Consciousness*
> *Is a fertile garden,*
> *Water it with the water of worship*
> *In the fullness of the action.*
> *Then, little by little, you will offer to the Shakti*
> *The fruits of this garden*
> *Where freedom will suddenly appear out of absolute nudity.*[13]

Here, this is simply about day, night, and sleep. Whether or not we practice dream yoga, as soon as we enter deeply into ourselves, presence is developed, and we participate in a sort of dreamlike revolution. First there is a chaotic fermenting process where dreams take on the utmost importance. This is both intense and disorderly. Then, when presence becomes established, dreams become milder and calmer, exactly as with presence to our actions. Sometimes we make an effort to slow down the action, but in reality, it is presence that makes the action slow down. When there is presence, the body begins to function differently. It can no longer function as before, in an intermittent manner. It is as if consciousness is gently emerging and the unfurling of the body is harmonizing itself with that consciousness.

Deep sleep is also pervaded by consciousness because once presence is established in dreams, we have the curious feeling that something is happening, whereas nothing is happening. We are neither in the waking state nor are we dreaming, nor are we in deep sleep. However, there is the continual sacred tremor, which we notice upon waking. Presence in dreams indicates to us that we have dreamed for a little while, and then that there was, between the end of the dream and the moment of waking, a period of time wherein something happened. We do not know exactly what, but the body has something to tell us. It is not an idea; it is not something mental that has come up: it truly is a feeling.

Usually we do not allow the body to speak. When the alarm clock rings, we jump out of bed, and two minutes later we are already engaged in frenetic activity. However, the moment of waking up is very important in the life of the tantrika because this is the moment when she gathers together everything that has happened in the unconscious. For this, all we have to do is be completely aware of the senses. Sometimes it is as if we are receiving abstract messages that we cannot translate and do not know what to do about. For a few minutes we realize we are receiving information that will influence the calmness of our day as well as our entry into activity. There is no rupture. It is not a different state. Everything is connected.

The presence of consciousness at the moment of emergence is simply the continuation of the experience. You will no longer feel at all that you are losing time in sleeping because sleep will have become a place of awareness. This will cause a deep intensity in continuous presence combined with a great lightness. Everything is very dense and completely airy. This comes simply from the continuity of experience throughout the three states. Little by little, reactivity stops in dreams themselves. Images may be terrifying, but you are no longer terrified. You let the film roll. You are conscious. You recognize the images as images. Agitation disappears.

STANZAS 26 AND 27

Mantras, when they are charged with the power of the
sacred tremor, accomplish their function through the
senses of the awakened person. They become united
with the mind of the tantrika, who penetrates the
nature of Shiva/Shakti.

Mantras emerge from the spatial source of the tantrika. They can have a form, or they can move toward formlessness. The formless mantra then becomes each sound of the universe, each vibration of the vocal cords, or of any other musical instrument. The person who is immersed in the source of consciousness is no longer anything but sacred tremoring. He has perfectly tuned the instrument of his body through the different yogas and takes pleasure in the absolute freedom of returning to the practice of living like a *sahajiya,* or spontaneous being, of being in permanent touch with his essence. This person then knows love and no longer fears death.

The goddess Tripura said:

> *The great mantra that I use is the intuition of my innate*
> *freedom.*[14]

⟨✦⟩

You can always tell yourself that in approximately mumbling some sounds you will bring about liberating forces. But you are dreaming. All you will produce is some "spiritual" noise. You will lose your breath, and your mouth will become dry. A yogin who knows how to use mantras can stop the sun, make the rain fall, paralyze, or kill. This has nothing to do with singing Boy Scout songs around the campfire. A mantra comes from silence. Attain silence first, and you will no longer need a mantra.

In the United States, gallons of mantric soup are produced, with little birds, synthesizers, and rivers. Walt Disney with a trident. Listen instead to the night, to the sounds of your body, to the unending interior dialogue that lives like a homeless squatter in the spatiality of your mind. If mantras really interest you, you will have to learn Sanskrit—the exact pronunciation, the music of each syllable—devote twenty or thirty years of your life to it with a master who knows the cosmic subtleties of this art. All the rest is only spiritual illusion.

However, if there is *spanda*, sacred tremoring, even a risky pronunciation can be powerful. The Pratyabhijna school is a sort of Tantric Ch'an. There are no accessories, no toys, no diversion, no romantic imaginings, no ideal, no hope. Instead, we go directly toward the reality of our functioning, toward our fear, our confusion, our perpetual hesitation, toward our violence, our jealousy, our hate, but also toward our original absolute splendor.

The absence of hope is not despair.* It is not that dreary and sad feeling, that apathy of the soul. It is, on the contrary, a state of opening to what is. It is the door to lightness, to spontaneity, and most of all, to

---

Translator's note: In French, the sense of polarity is more obvious. Hope is *espoir*; despair is *désespoir*.

fear being nearly over. Hope is masked fear seeking to reassure itself. When we get a glimpse, if only for a second, of the implications for the magic moment when we stop hoping, we reach space. We attain love.

Practicing without hope is very beautiful because we are not making anything up: we probe our interior, our consciousness, and our senses. All is meant for the recognition of our marvelous state. The idea of practicing meditation to obtain awakening leaves us, and everything becomes spontaneous. Spontaneity is of the utmost importance in the quest because it is the profound understanding that all of our capacities, ready to be unfurled, are waiting for us to recognize them. There is nothing in particular to do. We recognize everything in ourselves. The whole Tantric quest is directed inwardly by an awareness that fertilizes the latent traces. By considering the path in this manner, we will never be frustrated, never worried about the idea of not being true to ourselves. We will no longer keep incessantly thinking that we lack some refined qualities that we need in order to get to where everything is completely expressed. We will discover that there is nothing else to do but recognize. Everything begins to teem, to tremor, to establish connections. It is merely our ignorance of the essence that keeps us from attaining completeness. Once we turn our attention more deeply here, we discover all of these treasures. They emerge as if they have been waiting for centuries.

This is a beautiful way to see the human being. An enormous amount of confidence suddenly reigns between master and disciple, because the idea that one of them is going to do something for the other dies. Relationships become natural; there is no longer this expectation and waiting for something phenomenal on the part of the disciple who hopes to harvest a few bits of power from the master by watching him pass by or by touching the hem of his robe. There are two human beings. One helps the other only because he shows her that she is free and gives her the information that will allow her to make this extraordinary discovery on her own. Everything is there, marvelously present, ready to open and blossom. It is only a matter of giving oneself the space to acknowledge this power.

Self-Liberation through Seeing with Naked Awareness

Padmasambhava came from Odiyana, a neighboring kingdom of Kashmir. He brought the transmission of Mahamudra to Tibet in the eighth century of the common era and passed it on to his main disciple, Yeshé Tsogyal. He wrote this song:*

1   Here is contained "Self-Liberation through Seeing with Naked Awareness," this being a Direct Introduction to the State of Intrinsic Awareness, from "The Profound Teaching of Self-Liberation in the Primordial State of the Peaceful and Wrathful Deities."

2   Homage to the Trikaya and to the Deities who represent the inherent luminous clarity of intrinsic awareness.

3   Herein I shall teach "Self-Liberation through Seeing with Naked Awareness," which is a direct introduction to intrinsic awareness
From "The Profound Teaching of Self-Liberation in the Primordial State of the Peaceful and Wrathful Deities."
Truly, this introduction to your own intrinsic awareness
Should be contemplated well, O fortunate sons of a noble family!

SAMAYA gya gya gya!

4   Emaho!
It is the single (nature of) mind that encompasses all of Samsara and Nirvana.
Even though its inherent nature has existed from the very beginning, you have not recognized it.
Even though its clarity and presence has been uninterrupted,

---

*For an alternate translation, see Appendix 2, "The Natural Liberation through Naked Vision, Identifying Intelligence," translated by Robert A. F. Thurman.

you have not yet encountered its face.

Even though its arising has nowhere been obstructed, still you have not comprehended it.

Therefore, this (direct introduction) is for the purpose of bringing you to self-recognition.

Everything that is expounded by the Victorious Ones of the three times

In the eighty-four thousand Gateways to the Dharma

Is incomprehensible (unless you understand intrinsic awareness).

Indeed, the Victorious Ones do not teach anything other than the understanding of this.

Even though there exist unlimited numbers of scriptures, equal in their extent to the sky,

Yet with respect to the real meaning, there are three statements that will introduce you to your own intrinsic awareness.

This introduction to the manifest Primordial State of the Victorious Ones

Is disclosed by the following method for entering into the practice where there exists no antecedent nor subsequent practices.

5   *Kye-ho!*

O my fortunate sons, listen!

Even though that which is usually called "mind" is widely esteemed and much discussed,

Still it is not understood or it is wrongly understood or it is understood in a one-sided manner only.

Since it is not understood correctly just as it is in itself,

There come into existence inconceivable numbers of philosophical ideas and assertions.

Furthermore, since ordinary individuals do not understand it,

They do not recognize their own nature,

*And so they continue to wander among the six destinies (of
   rebirth) within the three worlds and thus experience suffering.*

*Therefore, not understanding your own mind is a very
   grievous fault.*

*Even though the Sravakas and the Pratyekabuddhas wish to
   understand it in terms of the Anatman doctrine,*

Still they do not understand it as it is in itself.

*Also there exist others who, being attached to their own
   personal ideas and interpretations,*

*Become fettered by these attachments and so do not perceive
   the Clear Light.*

*The Sravakas and the Pratyekabuddhas are (mentally)
   obscured by their attachments to subject and object.*

*The Madhyamikas are (mentally) obscured by their
   attachments to the extremes of the Two Truths.*

*The practitioners of the Kriya Tantra and the Yoga Tantra are
   (mentally) obscured by their attachments to seva-sadhana
   practice.*

*The practitioners of the Mahayoga and the Anuyoga are
   (mentally) obscured by their attachments to Space and
   Awareness.*

*And with respect to the real meaning of nonduality, since they
   divide these (Space and Awareness) into two, they fall into
   deviation.*

*If these two do not become one without any duality, you will
   certainly not attain Buddhahood.*

*In terms of your own mind, as is the case with everyone,
   Samsara and Nirvana are inseparable.*

*Nonetheless, because you persist in accepting and enduring
   attachments and aversions, you will continue to wander in
   Samsara.*

*Therefore, your active dharmas and your inactive ones both
   should be abandoned.*

However, since self-liberation through seeing nakedly by

means of intrinsic awareness is here revealed to you,
You should understand that all dharmas can be perfected and
completed in the great total Self-Liberation.
And therefore, whatever (practice you do) can be brought to
perfection within the Great Perfection.

SAMAYA gya gya gya

6   *As for this sparkling awareness which is called "mind,"*
Even though one says that it exists, it does not actually exist.
(On the other hand) as a source, it is the origin of the
diversity of all the bliss of Nirvana and all of the sorrow of
Samsara.

And as for its being something desirable, it is cherished alike
in the Eleven Vehicles.
With respect of its having a name, the various names that are
applied to it are inconceivable (in their numbers).
Some call it "the nature of the mind" or "mind itself."
Some Tirthikas call it by the name Atman or "the Self."
The Sravakas call it the doctrine of Anatman or "the absence
of a self."
The Chittamatrins call it by the name Chitta or "the Mind."
Some call it the Prajnaparamita or "the Perfection of
Wisdom."
Some call it the name Tathagatagarbha or "the embryo of
Buddhahood."
Some call it by the name Mahamudra or "the Great Symbol."
Some call it by the name "the Unique Sphere."
Some call it by the name Dharmadhatu or "the dimension of
Reality."
Some call it by the name Alaya or "the basis of everything."
And some simply call it by the name "ordinary awareness."

7   Now, when you are introduced (to your own intrinsic
       awareness), the method for entering into it involves three
       considerations:
     Thoughts in the past are clear and empty and leave no traces
       behind.
     Thoughts in the future are fresh and unconditioned by
       anything.
     And in the present moment, when (your mind) remains in its
       own condition without constructing anything,
     Awareness at that moment in itself is quite ordinary.
     And when you look into yourself in this way nakedly (without
       any discursive thoughts),
     Since there is only this pure observing, there will be found a
       lucid clarity without anyone being there who is the observer;
     Only a naked manifest awareness is present.
     (This awareness) is empty and immaculately pure, not being
       created by anything whatsoever.
     It is authentic and unadulterated, without any duality of
       clarity and emptiness.
     It is not permanent and yet it is not created by anything.
     However, it is not a mere nothingness or something
       annihilated because it is lucid and present.
     It does not exist as a single entity because it is present and
       clear in terms of being many.
     (On the other hand) it is not created as a multiplicity of things
       because it is inseparable and of a single flavor.
     This inherent self-awareness does not derive from anything
       outside itself.
     This is the real introduction to the actual condition of things.

8   Within this (intrinsic awareness), the Trikaya are inseparable
       and fully present as one.
     Since it is empty and not created anywhere whatsoever, it is
       the Dharmakaya.

*Since its luminous clarity represents the inherent transparent
    radiance of emptiness, it is the Sambhogakaya.*

*Since its arising is nowhere obstructed or interrupted, it is the
    Nirmanakaya.*

*These three (the Trikaya) being complete and fully present as
    one, are its very essence.*

9   *When you are introduced in this way through this exceedingly
        powerful method for entering into the practice,*

*(You discover directly) that your own immediate self-
    awareness is just this (and nothing else),*

*And that it has an inherent self-clarity that is entirely
    unfabricated.*

*How can you then speak of not understanding the nature of
    the mind?*

*Moreover, since you are meditating without finding anything
    there to meditate upon,*

How can you say that your meditation does not go well?

Since your own manifest intrinsic awareness is just this,

How can you say that you cannot find your own mind?

The mind is just that which is thinking;

*And yet, although you have searched (for the thinker), how
    can you say that you do not find him?*

*With respect to this, nowhere does there exist the one who is
    the cause of (mental) activity.*

*And yet, since activity exists, how can you say that such
    activity does not arise?*

*Since merely allowing (thoughts) to settle into their own
    condition, without trying to modify them in any way, is
    sufficient,*

*How can you say that you are not able to remain in a calm
    state?*

*Since allowing (thoughts) to be just as they are, without trying
    to do anything about them, is sufficient,*

How can you say that you are not able to do anything with
  regard to them?
Since clarity, awareness, and emptiness are inseparable and
  are spontaneously self-perfected,
How can you say that nothing is accomplished by your
  practice?
Since (intrinsic awareness) is self-originated and spontaneously
  self-perfected without any antecedent causes or conditions,
How can you say that you are not able to accomplish
  anything by your efforts?
Since the arising of discursive thoughts and their being
  liberated occur simultaneously,
How can you say that you are unable to apply an antidote?
Since your own immediate awareness is just this,
How can you say that you do not know anything with regard
  to it?

10   It is certain that the nature of the mind is empty and without
  any foundation whatsoever.
Your own mind is insubstantial like the empty sky.
You should look at your own mind to see whether it is like
  that or not.
Being without any view that decisively decides that it is
  empty,
It is certain that self-originated primary awareness has been
  clear (and luminous) from the very beginning,
Like the heart of the sun, which is itself self-originated.
You should look at your own mind to see whether it is like
  that or not.
It is certain that this primal awareness or gnosis, which is
  one's intrinsic awareness, is unceasing,
Like the main channel of a river that flows unceasingly.
You should look at your own mind to see whether it is like
  that or not.

*It is certain that the diversity of movements (arising in the
      mind) are not apprehensible by memories,*
*They are like insubstantial breezes that move through the
      atmosphere.*
*You should look at your own mind to see whether it is like
      that or not.*
*It is certain that whatever appearances occur, all of them are
      self-manifested,*
*Like the images in a mirror being self-manifestations that
      simply appear.*
*You should look at you own mind to see whether it is like
      that or not.*
*It is certain that all of the diverse characteristics of things are
      liberated into their own condition,*
*Like clouds in the atmosphere that are self-originated and
      self-liberated.*
*You should look at your own mind to see whether it is like
      that or not.*

11   *There exist no phenomena other than what arises from the
      mind.*
*Other than the meditation that occurs, where is the one who
      is meditating?*
*There exist no phenomena other than what arises from the
      mind.*
*Other than the behavior that occurs, where is the one who is
      behaving?*
*There exist no phenomena other than what arises from the
      mind.*
*Other than the samaya vow that occurs, where is the one who
      is guarding it?*
*There exist no phenomena other than what arises from the
      mind.*

Other than the fruition that occurs, where is the one who is realizing (the fruit)?
You should look at your own mind, observing it again and again.

12 *When you look upward into the space of the sky outside yourself,*
If there are no thoughts occurring that are emanations being projected,
And when you look inward at your own mind inside yourself,
If there exists no projectionist who projects thoughts by thinking them,
Then your own subtle mind will become lucidly clear without anything being projected.
Since the Clear Light of your own intrinsic awareness is empty, it is the Dharmakaya;
And this is like the sun rising in a cloudless illuminated sky.
Even though (this light cannot be said) to possess a particular shape 'or form, nevertheless, it can be fully known.
The meaning of this, whether or not it is understood, is especially significant.

13 *This self-originated Clear Light, which from the very beginning was in no way produced (by something antecedent to it),*
Is the child of awareness, and yet it is itself without any parents—amazing!
This self-originated primordial awareness has not been created by anything—amazing!
It does not experience birth nor does there exist a cause for its death—amazing!
Although it is evidently visible, yet there is no one there who sees it—amazing!

Although it has wandered throughout Samsara, it has come to no harm—amazing!

Even though it has seen Buddhahood itself, it has not come to any benefit from this—amazing!

Even though it exists in everyone everywhere, yet it has gone unrecognized—amazing!

Nevertheless, you hope to attain some other fruit than this elsewhere—amazing!

Even though it exists within yourself (and nowhere else), yet you seek for it elsewhere—amazing!

14   *How wonderful!*

This immediate intrinsic awareness is insubstantial and lucidly clear:

Just this is the highest pinnacle among all views.

It is all-encompassing, free of everything, and without any conceptions whatsoever:

Just this is the highest pinnacle among all meditations.

It is unfabricated and inexpressible in worldly terms:

Just this is the highest pinnacle among all courses of conduct.

Without being sought after, it is spontaneously self-perfected from the very beginning:

Just this is the highest pinnacle among all fruits.

15   *Here is the teaching of the four great vehicles that are without error:*

(First) there is the great vehicle of the unmistaken view.

Since this immediate awareness is lucidly clear,

And this lucid clarity is without error or mistake, it is called "a vehicle."

(Second) there is the great vehicle of the unmistaken meditation.

Since this immediate awareness is that which possesses clarity,

And this lucid clarity is without error or mistake, it is called "a vehicle."

(Third) there is the great vehicle of the unmistaken conduct.
Since this immediate primal awareness is that which possesses
   clarity,
And this lucid clarity is without error or mistake, it is called
   "a vehicle."
(Fourth) there is the great vehicle of the unmistaken fruit.
Since this immediate awareness is lucidly clear,
And this lucid clarity is without error or mistake, it is called
   "a vehicle."

16   *Here is the teaching on the four great unchanging (essential*
      points called) "nails."
(First) there is the great nail of the unchanging view:
This immediate present awareness is lucidly clear.
Because it is stable in the three times, it is called "a nail."
(Second) there is the great nail of the unchanging meditation:
This immediate present awareness is lucidly clear.
Because it is stable in the three times, it is called "a nail."
(Third) there is the great nail of the unchanging conduct:
This immediate present awareness is lucidly clear.
Because it is stable in the three times, it is called "a nail."
(Fourth) there is the great nail of the unchanging fruit:
This immediate present awareness is lucidly clear.
Because it is stable in the three times, it is called "a nail."

17   *Then, as for the secret instruction which teaches that the three*
      times are one:
You should relinquish all notions of the past and abandon all
   precedents.
You should cut off all plans and expectations with respect to
   the future.
And in the present, you should not grasp (at thoughts that
   arise) but allow (the mind) to remain in a state like the
   sky.

Since there is nothing upon which to meditate (while in the primordial state), there is no need to meditate.

And since there does not exist any distraction here, you continue in this state of stable mindfulness without distraction.

In this state, which is without meditation and without any distraction, you observe everything with a naked (awareness).

Your own awareness is inherently knowing, inherently clear, and luminously brilliant.

When it arises, it is called the Bodhichitta, "the enlightened mind."

Being without any activity of meditation, it transcends all objects of knowledge.

Being without any distraction, it is the luminous clarity of the Essence itself.

Appearances, being empty in themselves, become self-liberated; clarity and emptiness (being inseparable) are the Dharmakaya.

Since it becomes evident that there is nothing to be realized by means of the path to Buddhahood,

At this time you will actually behold Vajrasattva.

18   *Then, as for the instruction for exhausting the six extremes and overthrowing them:*

Even though there exist a great many different views that do not agree among themselves,

This "mind" which is your own intrinsic awareness is in fact self-originated primal awareness.

And with regard to this, the observer and the process of observing are not two (different things).

When you look and observe, seeking the one who is looking and observing,

Since you search for this observer and do not find him

At that time your view is exhausted and overthrown.

*Thus, even though it is the end of your view, this is the
    beginning with respect to yourself.*

*The view and the one who is viewing are not found to exist
    anywhere.*

*Without its falling excessively into emptiness and nonexistence
    even at the beginning,*

*At this very moment your own present awareness becomes
    lucidly clear:*

*Just this is the view (or the way of seeing) of the Great
    Perfection.*

*(Therefore) understanding and not understanding are not two
    (different things).*

19   *Although there exist a great many different meditations that
    do not agree among themselves,*

Your own ordinary present awareness is directly penetrating.

*The process of meditation and the one who meditates are not
    two (different things).*

*When you look for the meditator who is meditating or not
    meditating,*

*Since you have searched for this meditator and have not
    found him anywhere,*

At that time your meditation is exhausted and overthrown.

*Thus, even though it is the end of your meditation, this is the
    beginning with respect to yourself.*

*The meditation and the meditator are not found to exist
    anywhere.*

*Without its failing under the power of delusion, drowsiness,
    or agitation,*

*Your immediate unfabricated awareness becomes lucidly
    clear;*

*And this unmodified state of even contemplation is
    concentration.*

*(Therefore) remaining in a calm state or not remaining in it
are not two (different things).*

20   *Although there exist a great many different kinds of behavior
which do not agree among themselves
Your own self-originated primal awareness is the Unique
Sphere.
Behavior and the one who behaves are not two (different
things).
When you look for the one it is who behaves with action or
without action,
Since you have searched for the one who acts and have not
found him anywhere,
At that time your behavior is exhausted and overthrown.
Thus, even though it is the end of your conduct and behavior,
this is the beginning with respect to yourself.
From the very beginning neither behavior nor the one who
behaves have existed (as separate realities).
Without its falling under the power of errors and inherited
predispositions,
Your immediate awareness is an unfabricated inherent clarity.
Without accepting or rejecting anything, just letting things be
as they are without trying to modify them,
Such conduct or behavior alone is pure.
(Therefore) pure and impure action are not two (different things).*

21   *Although there exist a great many different fruits that do not
agree among themselves,
The nature of the mind that is inherent awareness is (none
other than) the spontaneously perfected Trikaya.
What is realized and the one who realizes it are not two
(different things).
When you look for the fruit and for the one who has realized it,
Since you have searched for the realizer (of the fruit) and have
not found him anywhere,*

At that time your fruit is exhausted and overthrown.

Thus, even though it is an end to your fruition, still this is the beginning with respect to yourself.

Both the fruition and the one who has attained the realization are found to not exist anywhere.

Without its falling under the power of attachments or aversions or of hopes and fears,

Your immediate present awareness becomes spontaneously perfected inherent clarity.

Understand that within yourself the Trikaya is fully manifest.

(Therefore) this itself is the fruition of primordial Buddhahood.

22   *This intrinsic awareness is free of the eight extremes, such as eternalism and nihilism, and the rest.*

Thus we speak of the Middle Way where one does not fall into any of the extremes

And we speak of intrinsic awareness as uninterrupted mindful presence,

Since emptiness possesses a heart that is intrinsic awareness,

Therefore it is called by the name of Tathagatagarbha, that is, "the embryo or heart of Buddhahood."

If you understand the meaning of this, then that will transcend and surpass everything else.

Therefore, it is called by the name of Prajnaparamita, that is, "the Perfection of Wisdom."

Because it cannot be conceived of by the intellect and is free of all (conceptual) limitations from the very beginning,

Therefore it is called by the name of Mahamudra, that is, "the Great Symbol."

Because of that, in accordance with whether it is specifically understood or not understood,

Since it is the basis of everything, of all the bliss of Nirvana and of all the sorrow of Samsara,

*Therefore it is called by the name of Alaya, that is, "the
foundation of everything."*
*Because, when it remains in its own space, it is quite ordinary
and in no way exceptional,*
This awareness that is present and lucidly clear
Is called by the name of "ordinary awareness."
*However many names may be applied to it, even though they
are well conceived and fancy sounding,*
*With regard to its real meaning, it is just this immediate
present awareness (and nothing else).*

23 *To desire something other than this*
*Is just like having an elephant (at home), but searching for its
tracks elsewhere.*
*Even though you may try to measure the universe with a tape
measure, it will not be possible to encompass all of it.*
*(Similarly) if you do not understand that everything derives
from the mind, it will not be possible for you to attain
Buddhahood.*
*By not recognizing this (intrinsic awareness for what it is),
you will then search for your mind somewhere outside of
yourself.*
*If you seek for yourself elsewhere (outside of yourself), how
can you ever find yourself?*
*For example, this is just like an idiot who, going into a crowd
of many people,*
*And having let himself become confused because of the
spectacle,*
*Does not recognize himself; and, even though he searches for
himself everywhere,*
*He continually makes the error of mistaking others for
himself.*
*(Similarly) since you do not see the natural condition of the
real disposition of things,*

*You do not know that appearances come from mind, and so
   you are thrust once again into Samsara.*

*By not seeing that your own mind is actually the Buddha,
   Nirvana becomes obscured.*

*With respect to Samsara and Nirvana, (the difference is simply
   due) to ignorance or to awareness respectively.*

*But at this single instant (of pure awareness), there is in fact
   no actual difference between them (in terms of their
   essence).*

*If you come to perceive them as existing somewhere other
   than in your own mind, this is surely an error.*

*(Therefore) error and nonerror are actually of a single essence
   (which is the nature of the mind).*

*Since the mind-streams of sentient beings are not made into
   something that is divided into two,*

*The unmodified, uncorrected nature of the mind is liberated
   by its being allowed simply to remain in its own (original)
   natural condition.*

*If you are not aware that the fundamental error or delusion
   comes from the mind,*

*You will not properly understand the real meaning of the
   Dharmata (the nature of reality).*

24   *You should look into what is self-arising and self-originated.*

*With respect to these appearances, in the beginning they must
   arise from somewhere,*

*In between they must remain somewhere, and at the end they
   must go somewhere.*

*Yet when you look (into this matter), it is, for example, like a
   crow gazing into a well.*

*When he flies away from the well, (his reflection) also departs
   from the well and does not return.*

In the same way appearances arise from the mind;

They arise from the mind and are liberated into the mind.

The nature of the mind which (has the capacity) to know
  everything and be aware of everything is empty and clear;
As is the case with the sky above, its emptiness has been
  inseparable from the very beginning.
Self-originated primal awareness becomes manifest,
And becoming systematically established as luminous clarity,
  just this is the Dharmata, the nature of reality.
Even though the indication of its existence is all phenomenal
  existence (which manifests externally to you),
You are aware of it in your own mind, and this latter is the
  nature of the mind.
Since it is aware and clear, it is understood to be like the sky.
However, even though we employ the example of the sky to
  indicate the nature of the mind,
This is in fact only a metaphor or simile indicating things in a
  one-sided fashion.
The nature of the mind, as well as being empty, is also
  intrinsically aware; everywhere it is clear.
But the sky is without any awareness; it is empty as an
  inanimate corpse is empty.
Therefore, the real meaning of "mind" is not indicated by the sky.
So without distraction, simply allow (the mind) to remain in
  the state of being just as it is.

25 *Moreover, as for this diversity of appearances, which*
  represents relative truth,
Not even one of these appearances is actually created in
  reality, and so accordingly they disappear again.
All things, all phenomenal existence, everything within
  Samsara and Nirvana,
Are merely appearances (or phenomena) which are perceived
  by the individual's single nature of the mind.
On any particular occasion, when your own (internal)
  mindstream undergoes changes,

*Then there will arise appearances, which you will perceive as
external changes.*

Therefore, everything that you see is a manifestation of mind.

*And, moreover, all of the beings inhabiting the six realms of
rebirth perceive everything with their own distinct karmic
vision.*

26   *The T'irthikas who are outsiders see all this in terms of the
dualism of eternalism as against nihilism.*

*Each of the nine successive vehicles sees things in terms of its
own view.*

*Thus, things are perceived in various different ways and may
be elucidated in various different ways.*

*Because you grasped at these various (appearances that arise),
becoming attached to them, errors have come into
existence.*

*Yet with respect to all of these appearances of which you are
aware in your mind,*

*Even though these appearances that you perceive do arise, if
you do not grasp at them, then that is Buddhahood.*

*Appearances are not erroneous in themselves, but because of
your grasping at them, errors come into existence.*

*But if you know that these thoughts only grasp at things that
are mind, then they will be liberated by themselves.*

Everything that appears is but a manifestation of mind

*Even though the entire external inanimate universe appears to
you, it is but a manifestation of mind.*

*Even though all of the sentient beings of the six realms appear
to you, they are but a manifestation of mind.*

*Even though the happiness of humans and the delights of the
Devas in heaven appear to you, they are but manifestations
of mind.*

*Even though the sorrows of the three evil destinies appear to
you, they are but manifestations of mind.*

Even though the five poisons representing ignorance and the
*   passions appear to you, they are but manifestations of mind.*
Even though intrinsic awareness, which is self-originated
*   primal awareness, appears to you, it is but a manifestation*
*   of mind.*
Even though good thoughts along the way to Nirvana appear
*   to you, they are but manifestations of mind.*
Even though obstacles due to demons and evil spirits appear
*   to you, they are but manifestations of mind.*
Even though the gods and other excellent attainments appear
*   to you, they are but manifestations of mind.*
Even though various kinds of purity appear to you, they are
*   but manifestations of mind.*
Even though (the experience) of remaining in a state of one-
*   pointed concentration without any discursive thoughts*
*   appears to you, it is but a manifestation of mind.*
Even though the colors that are the characteristics of things
*   appear to you, they are but manifestations of mind.*
Even though a state without characteristics and without
*   conceptual elaborations appears to you, it is but a*
*   manifestation of mind.*
Even though the nonduality of the one and the many appears
*   to you, it is but a manifestation of mind.*
Even though existence and nonexistence which are not created
*   anywhere appear to you, they are but manifestations of*
*   mind.*
There exist no appearances whatsoever that can be
*   understood as not coming from mind.*

27   *Because of the unobstructed nature of the mind, there is a*
*   continuous arising of appearances.*
Like the waves and the waters of the ocean, which are not
*   two (different things),*
Whatever arises is liberated into the natural state of the mind.

However many different names are applied to it in this
*   unceasing process of naming things,*
With respect to its real meaning, the mind (of the individual)
*   does not exist other than as one.*
And, moreover, this singularity is without any foundation and
*   devoid of any root.*
But, even though it is one, you cannot look for it in any
*   particular direction.*
It cannot be seen as an entity located somewhere, because it is
*   not created or made by anything.*
Nor can it be seen as just being empty, because there exists the
*   transparent radiance of its own luminous clarity and*
*   awareness.*
Nor can it be seen as diversified, because emptiness and
*   clarity are inseparable.*
Immediate self-awareness is clear and present.
Even though activities exist, there is no awareness of an agent
*   who is the actor.*
Even though they are without any inherent nature,
*   experiences are actually experienced.*
If you practice in this way, then everything will be liberated.
With respect to your own sense faculties, everything will be
*   understood immediately without any intervening operations*
*   of the intellect.*
Just as is the case with the sesame seed being the cause of the
*   oil and the milk being the cause of butter,*
But where the oil is not obtained without pressing and the
*   butter is not obtained without churning,*
So all sentient beings, even though they possess the actual
*   essence of Buddhahood,*
Will not realize Buddhahood without engaging in practice.
If he practices, then even a cowherd can realize liberation.
Even though he does not know the explanation, he can
*   systematically establish himself in the experience of it.*

(For example) when one has had the experience of actually tasting sugar in one's own mouth,

One does not need to have that taste explained by someone else.

Not understanding this (intrinsic awareness) even Panditas can fall into error.

Even though they are exceedingly learned and knowledgeable in explaining the nine vehicles,

It will only be like spreading rumors of places which they have not seen personally.

And with respect to Buddhahood, they will not even approach it for a moment.

If you understand (intrinsic awareness), all of your merits and sins will be liberated into their own condition.

But if you do not understand it, any virtuous or vicious deeds that you commit

Will accumulate as karma leading to transmigration in heavenly rebirth or to rebirth in the evil destinies respectively.

But if you understand this empty primal awareness which is your own mind,

The consequences of merit and of sin will never come to be realized,

Just as a spring cannot originate in the empty sky.

In the state of emptiness itself, the object of merit or of sin is not even created.

Therefore, your own manifest self-awareness comes to see everything nakedly.

This self-liberation through seeing with naked awareness is of such great profundity.

And, this being so, you should become intimately acquainted with self-awareness.

Profoundly sealed!

28   *How wonderful!*

As for this "Self-Liberation through Seeing with Naked
   Awareness," which is a direct introduction to one's own
   intrinsic awareness,

It is for the benefit of those sentient beings belonging to the
   later generations of those future degenerate times,

That all of my Tantras, Agamas, and Upadesas,

Though necessarily brief and concise, have been composed.

And even though I have disseminated them at the present
   time, yet they shall be concealed as precious treasures,

So that those whose good karma ripens in the future shall
   come to encounter them.

SAMAYA gya gya gya

This treatise which is an introduction to one's actual intrinsic
   awareness or state of immediate presence

Is entitled "Self-Liberation through Seeing with Naked
   Awareness."

It was composed by Padmasambhava, the Master from
   Uddiyana.

Until Samsara is emptied of living beings, may this Great
   Work of liberating them not be abandoned!

SARVA MANGALAM
PADMASAMBHAVA[15]

Third Flow
(Stanzas 28–52)

The Universal Nature Reflected in the Power of One's Own Nature

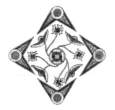

STANZAS 28 AND 29

All things emerge from the individual essence of the
tantrika who recognizes himself in Shiva/Shakti;
everything in which he takes pleasure is Shiva/Shakti.
Thus, there is no state that can be named that would
not be Shiva/Shakti.

In this inconceivable freedom, the spontaneous person sees in all manifestations only the glory of the Shiva/Shakti. Appearances, illusion itself, are nothing other than the divine, nothing other than consciousness. Wherever she turns, the tantrika is a worshipper of the divine within herself. The most infinitesimal part of the world conceals the totality of the universe. A speck of pollen is the cosmic beehive where the worshipper, like a bee, drunk on the beauty of the world, tastes the endless ambrosia that flows from all things.

Sahajanandabhairava sang:

> Whether I call it Mahamudra, Great Spatial Consciousness,
> Great Natural Perfection,
> Or Ch'an, the state of absolute union,
> I can neither conceive of it, nor pursue it, nor reach it.
> I can neither come closer to it nor get farther away from it
> Because it is the very nature of my mind.
> In this total nakedness,
> I abandon beliefs and concepts,
> Philosophies and certainties,
> All expectation and all fear.
> Then it comes forth from my depths.
> This is where it has always been.
> The Ruby of the Heart has only been waiting for
> My silence.
>
> What I would desire got farther away
> As I came closer to it.
> What I named would become unveiled,
> Effort would dry me up,
> Desire would make me like powder.
>
> The paradox of seeking is that we must
> Start seeking.
> But this, we find only by
> Abandoning seeking.
> Drifting in another place,
> I finally came back to the Heart.
> I have read a thousand descriptions of ambrosia

But I have tasted it only
By sipping of it myself.

I lost time wanting to probe the unknown,
To use up my wits,
I cluttered my consciousness.
Therefore, I separated myself from the known.

I crossed two spheres:
The sphere of accumulation
And the sphere of forgetting.
Finally I opened my senses to the inexpressible.
I realized that the absolute
Has no need for my theory of the world.
So I stopped obscuring the real.

I stopped opposing the concrete and the absolute,
Body and mind.
I stopped rambling on about the clouds
And finally I saw the sky.

Fragmentation maintained
Suffering and solitude.
In the great letting go,
Everything is luminous!
Glory be to the Goddess!
Glory be to my own absolute essence![1]

It is very reassuring to know that whatever we do, wherever we are, we will always be immersed in absolute essence. There is no different state, no place where we are separated from the essence. Nothing to do but continue to be totally present. This makes it possible to have intense union with all objects of desire. Once this discovery has been made, objects of desire are no longer different from ourselves. All is inner. As Abhinavagupta emphasizes, all desire is the reflection of the sole desire of the Self. Once we realize this, we no longer desire anything but the Self. Then all problems tied to desire are resolved. There is no state that can be named that would not be Shiva/Shakti. It is not worth the trouble of worrying about it. Let us flow with the current of the real, without expectation and without fear, without attachment and without detachment, in presence to the moment.

STANZA 30

Always present to the reality that he perceives as the
play of his own nature, the tantrika is liberated at the
very heart of life.

Immersed in ecstasy, the worshipper takes pleasure in the spatial freedom. Limitless, he contains the world. Open, struck by constant stupefaction, he travels gracefully and lightly through the planes of reality. The imaginary is peopled with rivers and mountains, nothing illusory; all thought creates an absolute reality, all emotion is the nectar from which the worshipper quenches his thirst. All is true, palpable, alive, tremoring. Silence itself is the symphony of all the sounds of the world together. Therefore, the worshipper no longer waits for anything; he escapes time; his body can disintegrate tranquilly in the space of ineffable reality.

Huang-po said:

> The absence of practice is my spiritual method, nothing other than the One Spirit. I ask you never to seek anything because what we seek, we lose in seeking it. Not to look for anything: this is tranquillity. Who told you to eliminate anything at all? Look at space!

How can you produce it or eliminate it? The only thing to do is to have no opinion at all. The mountains are the mountains, the rivers are the rivers; the earth, the mountains, the rivers, the ocean, the stars, are nothing other than your own heart.[2]

⁂

This perception that consciousness is the universe allows us to be both infinite and present to all the little details of life. That is, totally immersed in reality. We do not need to move into a cave or a monastery, because we already contain all that we are looking for outside of ourselves. This is truly the meaning of the practice: to enter into this creative dynamic where we let go completely in relation to the guilt of being, of doing, of doing too little, of succeeding or failing, of not being this or that, of having certain abilities and not others. We see little by little that all these abilities and all these limits are illusory in relation to our absolute essence, our original nature. Once we consider the whole of our functioning with love, there is blossoming.

Tantrism is a path where we learn to respect ourselves completely and to look at the extent to which our marvelous functioning and our innate freedom are hindered by our beliefs, our fears, our hope, our "spiritual" life. In experiencing freedom from time to time, all these micro-awakenings, suspended in space and interspersed with more or less difficult or chaotic periods, will become connected to each other and form a luminous and spatial network that will harvest each fleeting moment. From the time these moments of presence become part of our life, we enter into the practice of Mahamudra; but at the same time, we are doing absolutely nothing to practice, to collect spiritual experiences, to increase our "awakening capital." A vague act of presence occurs, and Mahamudra spreads everywhere. If we are tense, we do violence to ourselves. Practice can then become real aggression toward ourselves. A lot of seekers, obsessed with efficiency, get lost in this way. Once there is performance, it blocks us.

The Way is a game that consists of feeling that the only passionate thing in life is this vast abandoning to space, all the while giving to oneself the luxury of waiting for space and silence very gently to occur. When space and silence occur spontaneously, we will once again fall victim to frenzy. In the beginning, this works—indeed, quite well. We progress quickly; then suddenly everything disappears. Nothing further happens. Why? Because when intensity is excessive, we stop playing. We become a yogin with a mystical career plan. We predict our awakening in six months. We wonder if this will be the time of transmitting. We are already on hold. Our way is regressing to the source.

By maintaining the feeling of play, we can find the happy medium. We stop doing too much or too little about it. Our manner of practicing becomes refined, authentic. From time to time, a state emerges and we allow it to live, to go beyond, to lose itself.

STANZA 31

Through the intensity of objectless desire,
contemplation emerges in the heart of the tantrika
united to the profound sacred tremor.

The desire of the tantrika is never dampened—he is the sacred tremor itself, but he no longer goes through life like an arrow toward a target. He encircles all of reality like a halo, and in this space allows freedom to all trajectories. In this great cosmic movement of Mahamudra, the endless interlacings are the very blood of the tantrika. Like rainbow-colored ribbons, the different realities undulate endlessly in the sky of consciousness, which has recovered its true nature. The two schools of Pratyabhijna and Spanda are interconnected, and the intuitive sensing of our own original essence is all it takes to bring the Spanda into existence. This is the Great Natural Completeness. This is Mahamudra.

Tao-sin presented the five principles of nonpractice:

Recognize the essence of the mind. This essence is pure. It is identical to the Buddha.

Recognize the creativity of the mind. This creativity gives rise to the treasures of things whose emergence and functioning have always been peaceful, for all our distractions are manifestations of the essence.

Awakening is continual and never interrupted. The awakened consciousness unfurls before my eyes. The method of awakening is nonaspect.

Continual view of the emptiness and the peace of the body. Inner and outer are interpenetrated. The body slips into the very heart of the absolute domain and nothing can block it any more.

Maintain unity without deviating. The person who remains present, in movement as in stillness, sees clearly his Buddha nature and soon crosses the threshold of absorption.[3]

When we enter into the nonpractice of Mahamudra, the tremoring quality of desire no longer goes toward an object. Rather, it is desire itself that brings about the spatial peacefulness of the natural state. Everything under consideration in this text brings us back to leaving things in their natural state. There is nothing to reroute, nothing to transform. We are communicating with the reality of the various states of mind. Anger is anger, fear is fear, hope is hope. We are simply being present, understanding that this state is tranquillity. Once we are aware, we perceive that this desire, this sacred tremor, never stops. It is we who leave it. It is as if we are listening to musicians, and we go out of the room while the concert continues. This is presence: to remain listening to something that is in the process of happening. We might think that it is tiring to listen to this inner concert, but this is not true, because the musicians have the sensitivity to play pianissimo at times. This allows us to remain in the room, to hear the effects of the sounds, and to remain present to them. The beat becomes louder, softer, rises and falls, goes deeper or becomes infinitely light. All day long, we are animated by this coming and going of pulsation and the sacred tremoring that unfurls and remains always in the sphere of consciousness that is infinite freedom.

STANZA 32

This is the attainment of the supreme nectar, the immortality of samadhi, which reveals to the tantrika his own nature.

Eyes open on space, without blinking, the body relaxed, thought at rest, there no longer exists anything but ineffable reality flowing in the open space of our body, a vast mass grave where fertile chaos decomposes, where the yogin and the yogini love to stroll, their reflections crisscrossing: gods and goddesses, dakinis and dakas, dancing in the sky.

Sahajanandabhairava sang:

No hope, no needs, nothing lacking,
No projection, no expectations, no personal history,
No immobility. No movement,
No here, no elsewhere, the worlds are not divided.
Relax sensations, thought, and emotion,
Let them take their course spontaneously,
They become free like a cloud dissipating into space.
Taste of the limitless, because nothing is separated from your
   original essence.
Spacelike consciousness
Great fire of the Heart,
Indescribable joy at the heart of the Real.

Everything becomes free in the present moment.
Nothing to do or avoid,
Movement and stillness are luminous consciousness.
Free from seeking and from practice,
The essence of the heart inundates your whole being.
Your cosmic body is manifested in totality,
The cosmos tremors within your own dwelling-place!
Your voice resonates in the core of every atom,
Your gestures flow harmoniously,
This is spacelike nakedness!
The Land of the Heart! Mahamudra!
The essence of the most secret teachings!
May the vast portal of the sky open to infinity,
May your joy explode in a flow that nothing can impede,
May the infinite light of your body feed all people
In a gushing fountain of endless love!
The honey of this realization flows in every glitter of light,
Neither matter nor people are deprived of it,
The sun, the moon, the rocks, and the trees, the sky and the
*   earth,*
The body and the mind, do nothing but proclaim this Heart
*   vibrating to infinity!*[4]

Remember Tripura: She said that samadhi was the uninterrupted awareness of our own essence. When I would read the descriptions of samadhi, they would seem very mysterious to me. Then I saw yogins and yoginis in samadhi, and I started to get a sense of what this could be. Bottom line, samadhi is something that one can only know when one has "experienced" it (since experience no longer exists). Sometimes, if we are completely present and open, we enter into samadhi simply by looking at someone who is in this state. It is contagious. We do not know what is happening, but we suddenly feel that there is no separation, no longer duality.

If the text speaks of immortality, it is because at the moment when we enter into samadhi, we are not necessarily in a strange state. There are masters who are in uninterrupted samadhi and who continue to be involved in everyday life. The idea behind this is that when a person enters into this state, when a person is present to the totality of the sphere we are talking about in this text, both time and space cease to exist. We are in totality, and indeed sometimes we have trouble coming out of it. This can last for hours or days. The idea that samadhi is when a person leaves space-time has been present in Tantrism from its beginnings. It is an extremely profound experience that sometimes happens in unexpected ways, when we are not in the middle of practicing or meditating. (By the way, no one has ever attained awakening while meditating, but always when face to face with the real. Even the Buddha experienced awakening at the *end* of his meditation when he saw the morning star.)

When we enter into samadhi due to our master being in samadhi, it is as if we are receiving the gift of the experience before we have the means to enter into it. Strangely we are overtaken by a state that we know nothing about, even if we have read all the texts about it. Concepts crumble; expectations are completely shaken up by the space that pervades us. It is a very sweet state. There is nothing other than unbelievable, luminous presence. It can last a few minutes, or more. We might believe that in order to enter it, we must go through something violent or very powerful. No, it is a gentle explosion that scares us because we lose all support, all points of reference, all known dimensions. Escaping from the known, we enter into a dimension that is now neither space nor time: the infinite.

On the path, we often seek to reach states that we already know, and this is normal. But this seeking quickly blocks us: We imagine states, we dream of certain things, and one day we reach them, we realize what we have imagined—we realize something minuscule, invented, artificial, which we take for the infinite. The day that our fantasies materialize—which always happens—then we enter into a period of stagnation that can be very long. When I first would enter into samadhi in the presence of Kalu Rinpoche or Devi, it was as if their presence were pulling me toward the state manifested by their heart of spatiality. Later, when I was capable of putting myself in this state on my own, I started to play with it, putting myself into samadhi every chance I got. Devi told me not to do this. She said that it was not a game, that my practice was becoming vulgar, that I needed to wait until it happened by itself.

Samadhi is a grace. It is not a commodity. This is very difficult because once our body has registered how it works—the stillness, the quasi-absence of breathing, as if the skin were breathing—we try to reproduce it. Then samadhi becomes artificial, and very quickly it becomes confinement. What is important is to not induce a state, even if it is pleasant. If we do this, the quest tightens up completely. As a master from the past would say, we end up like a rat caught in a pipe that grows narrower and narrower. Every time Devi saw me creating samadhi she would interrupt me on purpose, until finally, no longer seeking it, I experienced the surprise of grace.

When we no longer make any effort to produce such and such a state, our experience becomes very interesting because it is always different. When each experience is a discovery, at this point we truly escape from the known. In this way we avoid the biggest trap, that of repeating the experience through breathing techniques or by abandoning techniques. If we allow this state to overtake us, we have the impression that there are hundreds of different samadhis. What is wonderful in the quest is finding a form of independence in the act of making something up. By allowing matters to happen on their own, we find the continuous freshness of not waiting for anything in particular, and we see the gifts coming freely.

This stanza encourages us to overcome automatic and mechanical response in order to discover wonderment. Something happens that is neither predicted nor awaited. Then we know spontaneous wonderment, an opening of the heart.

STANZAS 33 AND 34

The ardor toward Shiva/Shakti that manifests the
universe allows the tantrika to be fulfilled. Over the
course of the dream, the sun and the moon appear in
his heart and all his wishes are granted.

The tantrika then discovers that only the blaze of ardor is required, and
that all forms, all rituals, all practices are only aspects of divine play, of
the creativity of Shiva/Shakti. Then there is nothing to do but abandon
oneself to the great fire of/in the heart where the sun and the moon
touch lips and, in the midnight blue sky, are united both night and day
in the reality of the dream, and in the dream of Reality.

Mazu:
> *All matters are matters of the Heart*
> *All names are names of the Heart*
> *Everything comes from the Heart*
> *Everything has as its source the Heart.*[5]

Huang-po:
> *Finding nothing to transmit is what is called transmitting the*
> *Heart. The Buddha and people are one and the same*
> *Heart. There is no other reality.*[6]

In the *Lankavatarasutra:*
> *All things are only the Heart.*[7]

Bodhidharma:
> *The Heart itself is the Buddha, the Buddha is the Heart.*
> *Outside of the Heart, there is in the end no Buddha that*
> *one can obtain.*[8]

Sahara sang:

> *When your Heart is freed from thought, you are now only*
> *one with the Guru.*[9]

Fieriness toward Shiva/Shakti is fieriness in regard to our own potential—because the potential of Shiva/Shakti is within us. This fieriness encourages things to open and blossom. This is worship, *bhakti*. Often we believe that it is devotion toward Shiva/Shakti, but devotion is something that we can feel toward our own absolute possibilities, the master of which can be the mirror in which they are reflected. We then see with wonderment that all aspects of the divine are within us. This wonderment brings about a sweetness that is the prelude to the sacred tremor, to samadhi, to a complete opening. Then experiences become intense, they last longer, and it is difficult to come out of them, even when making an effort to do so. In this state of profound presence, all can happen without coming out of the state. Samadhi is not something to preserve by keeping oneself isolated in a secret hiding place. It is something that can occur for a few hours or a few days, then slowly diminishes until it disappears only to return later, spontaneously.

STANZA 35

But if he is not present, the tantrika will be wronged by
the play of manifestation, and he will experience the
illusory state of the aspirant throughout waking and
sleeping.

Absence from the world is almost the same as presence. The only difference is that the divine game seems like fate, whereas the yogin and the yogini, made alert by the extreme sensitivity of their bodies, taste each emergence as an offering that Shiva/Shakti make to the worshipper of their own immaculate essence.

Foyan:

> *Those who realize the awakening of Chan transcend subject and object. Besides this, there is no other mysterious principle.*[10]

When we have reached the sphere of ecstatic presence, we will see it like a somewhat magical state, and we will tend to use it like a drug. In other words, lulled within this state of happiness, our presence will diminish, and we will quickly come to live in a false kind of wonderment, as if it were caused by some drug. Extraordinary or magical occurrences will take place, but we will not have this profound presence, this sharpness. We will fall victim to an illusion. This is why the Ch'an master Yuanwu advised his disciples to dispose of marvels and mysteries like so much garbage, and why Devi found the yogins or the masters who performed "miracles" extremely vulgar. As marvelous as they might be, they are only obstacles on the path.

This is one of the important points where the presence of a master is indispensable. He is there to put a stop to all the states that we think we have attained. He replaces stopping places with space—a certainty of realization with a shout or a burst of laughter—until the great letting go, when we no longer need the master to hand us a certificate of authenticity. At that point, the master smiles; we have recognized our identity, and we are one with him and with totality.

Even samadhi plunges us back into the ego, making us lose all the benefits of what we have experienced. However, there is a moment when all these experiences become so fluid that they approach the indefinable. And when we are no longer sure of the state we were in, our practice truly becomes a deep practice. We no longer need to label the states, by which we risk becoming a sort of mystical catalog of cheap, junky trinkets. In all stages of the quest, each time that we have an experience, we must tell ourselves that it is magnificent, that it is a gift, but that it is not necessarily something to do again, to try to find again. This gives us great freedom on the path and leads us toward the most varied perceptions—because we no longer have this attachment, nor this pride in having arrived, in having succeeded. The quest knows no end.

We will then freely experience the passages, the movement, the wave, the highs and lows, openings and closings as movement. And movement is the fundamental aspect of yoga, the freedom of a river that follows its course toward the ocean and does not conceptualize the meandering, the flooding, the droughts, the widening, or the arrival at the vast space it finally will pour into.

STANZAS 36 AND 37

Just as an object that escapes attention is more clearly
perceived when we make the effort to see it better
from all angles, so the supreme sacred tremor appears
to the tantrika when he ardently strives toward it. In this
way, everything is in tune with the essence of his true
nature.

The effort to understand from all angles is the abandonment of limits, the letting go of the body-mind. Then the great fluctuation is established, we hear ourselves, and we come back toward our center without ever leaving the original source. Every point of the movement then becomes immensity itself, and the wave of the Real does not find its fall dizzying, nor its ascension fleeting as it breaks into silver foam in the space of the sky.

Pao-tche:

There is no treasure besides a luminous pearl
In the Heart of this body.[11]

Tripura:

> *It is passion for deliverance that is the principal means of
> salvation, and it is the man animated by this passion who is
> the true believer. The way to reach supreme deliverance is
> to desire it passionately. To believe that this passion has
> become total and exclusive: no other means is required.*[12]

It is a simple experience. If we look distractedly at a candle, we will be unaware of its reality. If we look at it a second time with a little more presence, we start to see a great many details: the quality of the flame, the edge of the wax, its transparency, the color, the inside. Little by little, we become the candle. In the quest, we must try to maintain at the same time true ardor and detachment in that ardor, to feed this fieriness with a lot of subtlety, sensitivity, and lightness. If we hang onto the creative surge, we cannot reproduce the experience. This fieriness gives us the desire to create continually, all the while being completely relaxed toward the object. We are then carried toward something indefinable. We invent as we go along. We truly know wonderment because there is never repetition. Repetition engenders stagnation, tightening, death. And when we speak of the contraction of the Shakti, this points exactly to this desire to repeat things that are unique.

STANZA 38

Even in a state of extreme weakness, such a tantrika
succeeds in this accomplishment. Even starving, he
finds his food.

When the body moves toward the great and ultimate relaxation, the nature of space is even more perceptible to us because the energy of action is at its weakest level. Now nothing veils absolute Reality any more, and our mouth becomes the mouth of the yoginis, ours the heart of the yoginis, the yoni of the yoginis into which we melt in space, where we rightly belong.

Jayratha:

> *The universal Heart is identical to the Ultimate Reality, to the vibration of Consciousness, and to the acquiring of global Consciousness of the absolute "I," the Heart of the yoginis.*[13]

This is a stanza directed against those who claim that if one does not die harmoniously, one will experience terrifying reincarnations. This obsession was very strong at the time this text was written—and it remains so to this day! Most people are terrified at the idea of dying senile or of having a violent or sudden death. They have the impression that if their death is stolen from them, gone will be the possibility of moving on to something else that exists beyond. This creates a kind of terror in everyone, and even more so in people following a spiritual path, who are often irreparably affected by theist and eternalist concepts. Their greatest desire is to have a peaceful and progressive death. But it does not happen like that. Most people die in the hospital or in unforeseeable and tragic circumstances. Tantric masters have said that all of this is unimportant, and that from the moment we are in opening, even if we take complete leave of our senses, we preserve our innate spatiality. This is a very beautiful stanza because it rids us of the guilt feelings associated with worrying about dying badly and permits us, should the circumstances be difficult, to be unafraid of what will happen to us.

This is meaningful when we stay with people who are dying. Often their state is not wonderful and their awareness is limited. We worry for ourselves and sometimes for them. But if we understand in a deep way that this is not at all important, we will be present to their death in a much gentler way. And we can help them, since we no longer feel apprehension for them. Even if we cannot talk with them or they cannot hear us, we can help, because we are carrying them within us; they are resting in our tranquillity. We know that, despite their state, their consciousness can emerge completely, and perhaps they can hear very well what we have to communicate when they are crossing through that moment.

STANZA 39

With his only support the recognition of the heart, the tantrika is omniscient and in harmony with the world.

Recognition of the heart is Mahamudra, the state of cosmic consciousness, the instantaneous return to the source of the original mind, where nothing is divided. In this unity, there is only harmony. All seeking makes us believe that the infinite is outside of us, and a dynamic is created to find a place of peace that does not exist outside of the heart. When this confusion-producing energy fades away, what happens is the great return of the mind to its natural state. There is nothing to find outside of this, and all the secret teachings do nothing other than establish this fundamental truth. Leaving consciousness in order to find consciousness is the great tragedy of the spiritual search. The end of all seeking coincides with the attainment of harmony, joy, and tranquillity.

The great master Padmasambhava sang the song of the ultimate practice:
In the Mind free from concepts:
Remain in equalness, with no meditation.
Even (if you) meditate, remain naturally, with no negating.
Remain in instantness, with no wavering,
Even if you waver, remain freely, with no negating.
Remain in suspension, with no watching.

Even (if you) watch, remain blank, with no negating.
Remain in instinctiveness, with no projecting.
Even if you project, remain "herely," with no negating.
Remain in distinctiveness, without withdrawing.
Even (if you) withdraw, remain clearly, with no negating.
Remain in openness, with no exertions.
Even (if you) exert, remain restrained, with no negating.
Remain in lucidity, with no modifications.
Even (if you) modify, remain purely, with no negating.
Remain in effortlessness, with no acquiring,
Even if you (acquire), remain spontaneously, with no
  negating.
Remain in spontaneity, with no rejecting.
Even (if you) reject, remain in the unborn, with no negating.
Remain in alertness, with no limits.
Even (if you) are limited, remain naturally, with no negating.
Remain in relaxation, with no efforts.
Even (if you) make efforts, remain spontaneously, with no
  negating.
Remain in no-basis, with no contemplation.
Even (if you) contemplate, remain spontaneously, with no
  negating.[14]

This stanza rids of us of the guilt of the idea that we must amass theo-
retical knowledge in order to enter into deep mystical states. Kallata
tells us that, with the recognition of the heart as sole support, we will
succeed. We can leave texts and knowledge aside. Certain masters, after
a certain point, keep their disciples from reading anything at all and
teach them extremely simple things like breathing and abandoning the
body to space through the dance of Shiva, our yoga, tantra yoga. Our
curiosity is legitimate—on the condition that it not be considered the
essential part. Then we can relax completely concerning accumulation
and the desire to make a performance of our knowledge of philosophy.

If we aspire simply to be present, to be conscious of our breath, we can do without all the rest, and we can even stop reading completely.

When we experience a state of nonduality, we are at the very source from which all the mystical texts emerge. We no longer need books. We know their contents through our own experience. Of course, we can both experience the source and read books, but the source liberates us from the voracious attitude that we have toward books. I have practiced intellectual voracity a lot—which is why I am speaking to you about it here. And one day I realized that it was completely useless. Yet I still had this desire to read everything that was published on the subjects that interested me. I even ordered books from India, Japan, and China. Let us not forget that realization is completely independent of anything whatsoever, especially books.

STANZA 40

If the body/mind is ravaged by discouragement due to ignorance, only the completely unlimited expansion of consciousness will dissipate a lassitude whose source will then have disappeared.

Man endlessly crosses the deserts looking for his eyes outside of his head. He sees the mountains and the lakes, the rivers and the forests, the shimmering light, the celestial canopy and the blue sky, the stars and the Milky Way; but, not finding his eyes, he grows weary. He is overcome with fatigue. He ends up losing his sight. Suddenly, he can no longer see anything and, in this very darkness, he realizes that the mountains and the rivers, the sky and space are in his own heart. When he opens his eyes again, he sees that all that previously seemed outside of him now shimmers and vibrates in his own heart. He is overcome with joy. Finally, he sees.

Yuanwu explains Mahamudra in his letter entitled "The Secret Seal":

Here at my place, there is no Zen to explain and no Path to transmit. Though five hundred patched-robed ones [monks] are gathered together here, I just use the diamond trap *and the* thicket of thorns. . . .

In essence, you cannot find where this one comes from: it's called the fundamental matter that is inherent in everyone. As soon as you deliberately intend to accept it or take it up, this is already not the fundamental anymore. Just get the myriad impulses to cease, so even the thousand sages do not accompany you—then how could there still be any dependency?

You should put everything aside right away and penetrate through to freedom on that side. That is why it is said, "Even the slightest thing is dust—as soon as you rouse your intellect you are assailed by the demons of delusion."

Forming all things just depends on that; *destroying all things also just depends on* that.

What should be formed and perfected? The causal conditions of special excellence, the treasury of merits and virtues countless as the sands, the countless wondrous adornments and world-transcending rarities.

What should be destroyed and obliterated? Greed and anger and jealousy, emotional consciousness and attachments, contrived actions and defiled actions, filth and confusion, names and forms and the interpretive route, arbitrary views and knowledge and false sentiments.

That transforms all things, but nothing can transform that. *Though it has no shape or visage, it contains all of space. It contains the ordinary and nurtures the holy. If you try to grasp it through forms, then in grasping at it, you fall into the thorns of views, and you will never find it.*

It was just this wondrous mind that the buddhas revealed and the ancestral teachers directly pointed out. When you take it up directly, without producing a single thought, and penetrate from the heights to the depths, everything appears ready-made. Here where it appears ready-made, you do not exert any mental effort: you go along freely with the natural flow, without any grasping or rejecting. This is the real esoteric seal.[15]

Discouragement and weariness are fruitful moments. They represent a natural pause that comes along to interrupt the course of our eagerness. The cessation of a dynamic carries space within itself. The guilty feeling of our incapacity can lead us to despair, and despair can lead us to silence and joy—provided that we dare to remain there, to settle in there, in some way. In the end of hope exists the seed of the end of fear, the smell of freedom and independence. Let us dare to abandon the frenzy of seeking. Let us dare to stand aloof, to doubt all that has seemed essential to us up until now, let us dare to stop believing in anything at all; then we will have the experience of a great letting go. Then, in this relaxing, we will perhaps be able to taste of the essence of inconceivable freedom.

STANZA 41

The revelation of the Self arises in the person who is now only absolute desire. May each of us have this experience!

Thus is born absolute desire, the intuitive sense of the energy of love, the passionate worship of the real. The worshipper finally finds the treasure in her own dwelling place. The Ruby of the Heart was so close that, by turning her gaze toward herself, she finally sees it. This realization does not require a gradual path, an apprenticeship, the usage of forms and rituals, yoga, and asceticism. Only absolute desire is indispensable, the inward gaze.

Niu-tou said:

There is no place that is not the Way![16]

Jayaratha sang:

Those who preceded us taught that we end desire by practicing detachment. We teach that this can be attained by abstaining from all effort.[17]

Since the beginning of this text, we have been talking about absolute desire. That is, incandescence carried by itself and not by the object of desire. This energy shakes us up, disturbs us, and pushes us toward the infinite. It is this incandescence that allows us, even if an object has triggered it, little by little to dissolve it—the object—in absolute love, non-neurotic love, love empty of sentimentality but not of feeling. The object will not disappear for all that, but the passion it released will suddenly explode and be submerged by the blossoming of absolute desire. What changes in life is our relationship to this object, now integrated with the fullness of the Self. From the moment we experience this outburst, we rediscover the object of desire in all things. It becomes omnipresent and without characteristics. In a certain sense, it no longer exists as a separate entity. We reach in this way a state beyond frustration. There is this magnificent and continual presence.

This is what happens when we have a deep relationship with a master who gives us the key to neurotic detachment and has us taste the insane effervescence of objectless love. At first we are tied to him; later, we are tied to everything; and then we reach fundamental freedom. We cannot forget him because he is within us. We no longer feel the imperial need to see him physically because he resides in each of our cells and lives, beyond life and death, in our heart. We are no longer obsessed with the idea of being with him—because we never leave him. One cannot speak about one's dead master in the past. He is just as we are: beyond time and space. So, if it happens, it is wonderful, and if it doesn't, that is wonderful too—because in our absolute solitude is the key to our freedom. This incandescence is the great Tantric secret!

STANZA 42

Then, may light, sound, form, and taste come and
impede the person who is still tied to the ego.

When the inner gaze opens, sounds do nothing but caress the absolute substance of things, and the ego loosens to the point where it becomes the Self.

Chen-houei said:
> *How can one call the act of disciplining the mind*
> *"deliverance"?*[18]

This is for the person who has not understood the preceding stanza. Poor him! Hindered, tied hand and foot, in total paralysis! And yet even this hindering, if we live it completely, is the key to our liberation. The senses kill us or liberate us. The sensorial quest can be the tragic site of illusion—or the expression of the divine within us. Do the gods know this inconceivable freedom? Do we know it? Here again is an opportunity for healthy doubt. Why did we create the gods?

STANZA 43

When the tantrika pervades everything with his
absolute desire, what use are words? He has this
experience on his own.

Finally, silence settles in, the yogin and yogini reside there, and desire palpitates within like the energy of love. Everything manifested comes rushing into the heart of those who are inhabited by this absolute desire. Rain and snow fall in the heart, the sun and the moon make their way across the heart, rainbows unfurl in the limitless space of the body.

Vimalakirti said:
> *The Real cannot be compared to anything since it is absolute.*
> *The throne of awakening is joy that takes pleasure in the*
> *Real. Awakening is the result because one keeps oneself at*
> *the summit of the Real.*[19]

Mazu:
> *I teach Reality![20]*

What use are words? The energy of sounds and language are related to the garland of letters. The yoga of the garland of letters is a very interesting practice. Abhinavagupta wrote a whole text on this subject and said that making use of it consists of deconstructing language. There also exists a Tantra that is wholly dedicated to the garland of letters. It is a minuscule, meticulous study of what happens through language, of the how and the why of our connection to words, of how the mind works with images and the words we use.

To practice this yoga, we focus our attention on the words and letters, and we dissolve them in space. This work is done with common
sentences that come up, and in general sentences that are connected to
beliefs: "I am Tantric, I believe in the immaculate essence, I believe in
reality, I believe in the illusion of all things, I believe in consciousness,
in the Self, in the divine integrated with the Self, and in all the logical
stages of the advance toward completeness. I believe in nonseparation.
I believe in nonduality, in spatiality, in freedom, and in all the didactic
twaddle used by tradition." By entering into phonemes, the person
makes them explode and reaches space. A whole part of the
Vijnanabhairava Tantra addresses this practice.

STANZA 44

May the tantrika remain present, his senses vigilantly
sown in reality, and may he know stability.

In presence is found the spontaneous meditation of Mahamudra. This
is why we speak of nonmeditation. Nothing to do, nothing to elabo-
rate, nothing to seek: everything flows naturally from the essence of
the mind. When the tension of the mind that is brought on by the ego
ceases, duality collapses, and we taste the unique flavor of all things.
In this great abandon lies the secret that no one believes in because it
is of a revolting simplicity. It is the negation of all the paths, of all
ascendancy over people, of all hope, of all trajectory. The Ruby of the
Heart is manifested within you in this instant. Nothing can veil or
obscure it.

Trungpa said:
    The absence of struggle is in itself liberation.[21]

Stability is an exhilarating state that is tied to the real. No longer anything contained, no longer anything mental. The body explodes toward the unlimited. What more is there to say?

STANZA 45

The person who is deprived of his power by the dark forces of limited activity becomes the plaything of the energy of sounds.

Therefore, without giving yourself over to the energy of action that goes about always seeking something like a roaming dog looking for food, do not let yourself go toward illusion because, if you do, you will become the plaything of the dark energy and forces. You are what you seek. Your essence is immaculate, perfect, it is the Great Completeness, Mahamudra.

Niu-tou said:

> Do not destroy the emotions of common people;
> Only teach them the cessation of thoughts.[22]

Let us stop acting . . . truly . . . radically . . . definitively!

STANZAS 46, 47, AND 48

Caught in the field of subtle energies and mental
representations, the supreme ambrosia is dissolved,
and the person forgets his innate freedom.

The power of the word is always ready to veil the
profound nature of the Self because no mental
representation can free itself from language.

The energy of the sacred tremor that passes through
the vulgar person enslaves him, whereas this same
energy liberates the person who is on the path.

When we direct our powerfulness outwardly, we fall into the nets of
mental representations, we create limited objectives, and then we seek
to attain them—thereby losing the memory itself of original completeness. Words, teachings, viewpoints, all come along to enchain us always
more tightly to the limited. Everything is adulterated by the mental
processes, which instantaneously transform the absolute teaching into
an object to be seized. And the teaching of Mahamudra cannot be
seized; it can only emerge from our own heart in the grace and the lightness of total abandon.

In the *Nirvana Sutra:*
> *Space can contain everything, but space has no concept of the*
> *thought that it can contain everything.*[23]

Here we have another stanza that addresses the energy of words, of speech, and of automatic internal talk. For centuries, we stopped talking about this in the West, but it was already known by the yogis thousands of years ago. In other words, internal talk, present every second, conditions us unendingly. What is interesting when we practice is to observe how we think, and whether we think without using words—in images, for example. Each time that you are in the process of thinking, try to see what is the connection to words. Quite obviously, we talk internally. We mutter all day long. The practice of this yoga consists of becoming conscious of this drivel, and awareness finally stops it. We can have a direct relationship with the Self and no longer with this hodgepodge of words. Let us seek to shed light on them from the inside until the time comes when they vanish into space.

When we succeed in entering into moments of consciousness, our success does not come from academic formulations and guilt-provoking discourse. There is a very different kind of presence: no guilt, no philosophy, no mysticism! It no longer passes through this sort of electronic translation. It seems a step is missing, as if between the experience and the person who experiences it, suddenly the filter of language no longer exists. The filters are clogged with language. If we succeed, even if only for a few seconds, we develop presence, even toward language, because in an underlying way, the intensity of the direct experience is present.

This is a powerful yoga, especially for those of us who have a fast-paced mental system that turns quickly, going over and over things endlessly, to the point of a madness. The practice allows us to find spaces where all sensations are there, but there no longer exists this second version of reality. Automatic thought is but a sorry photocopy of a photocopy of the Real where everything is illusory. There is no illusion.

STANZAS 49 AND 50

The subtle body itself is an obstacle that is tied to
limited intelligence and to the ego. The enslaved
person has experiences that are tied to his beliefs and
to the idea that he has of his body, and in this very way
perpetuates the tie.

The division of the bodies, their spatial distinction, creates duality. There is only this unlimited body that is neither large nor small, neither physical nor spatial. It is totality, and everything that emerges flows within it. The gods and the goddesses make their home of it; this body is the jewel of the limitless; it transcends all views and all yogas. Without the help of practice, it glimmers until infinity, and all the experiences on which aspirants pride themselves are nothing but thought made rigid by illusion. Hence, abandon all image of your destination, and your journey toward the Ruby of the Heart will be free of obstacles. To attain what you seek is the illusion that the demons hold out to you. To find what you seek is to get stuck in your own trap. Free yourself from the goal, free yourself from attaining, and Mahamudra will occur in its sparkling clarity.

Abhinavagupta said:

> The Heart is called the resting place of the immaculate light
> and of Pure Consciousness, which is not different from all
> the parts of the body.[24]

During interviews or questions, those who believe in certain things say that they are sure it is this way because they have experienced it. Not for a second do they see that their experience is caused by their belief.

This is obviously something very subtle. This stanza is a little dig at the intentions of traditional yoga, where there is much discussion on different forms of the body. Here, it is simply being said that when one believes that the subtle body exists, one will have an experience of the subtle body; when one believes that a bicycle created the universe, one will have mystical dreams about the bicycle that created the universe and the stigmata of a cyclist. This is therefore a key for taking inventory of our beliefs and for seeing how those experiences that confirm certain beliefs are tied to our certainties. This is something extraordinary—it deconditions us from certainty and leads us into this very Tantric domain where nothing is affirmed and nothing is denied. Then we save an extraordinary amount of energy that we can use in the real work. We no longer have this necessity to cling to beliefs and dogmas, nor to deny them: We are free. We can simply enter into the reality of the body, thoughts, sensations.

Now, each time we have an experience that seems to confirm a notion, even an uncertain one, we will continue to cling to it, but with a little smile on our lips—because we know that we are having an experience of what we believe. It is a subtle observation, as we are used to reasoning in the other direction, where we live our experiences as proof of our beliefs. It is important to do this with our little daily beliefs as well. For tantrikas, this is play. We construct something, then take apart the thing constructed, and this leads us to spatiality.

We never have the idea that a construction is made to be definitive; rather, we see it as a cycle of appearances and disappearances. We create a vision, and we reabsorb it by attention to the vacuity that disappears in plenitude and joy. When we do lineage yoga, it is exactly the same. We create something from start to finish, we put it into vibration, and then we allow it to unmake itself in light, in vibrating darkness. At the end of the practice, we get a taste of space.

STANZA 51

But when the tantrika becomes established in the
sacred tremor of reality, he liberates the flow of
manifestation and return, and in this way takes pleasure
in the universal freedom, as a master of the wheel of
energies.

So, absolute freedom spontaneously gushes forth like a spring. Nothing comes along to limit the yogin and the yogini, the flow and the sacred tremor are infinite, the wheel of energies is set into motion, and the gods and goddesses come to pay homage to the person who has attained these miraculous powers. His body is integrated into space, and Mahamudra occurs in completeness. The Ruby of the Heart shines forever, and the people are illuminated.

Houei-neng said:

The way is but communication and fluidity.[25]

This stanza brings us back to the first, that is, that the tantrika will experience within himself the divine state of creation and reabsorption that was attributed to the Shakti at the beginning of the text, and he will know that the gods are merely the Self. This is the manifestation of all the symbolism attached to divinity. It is this power of creation and reabsorption itself, which is inside of the consciousness of the yogin, that causes the cycle to end in universal freedom. As for the wheel of energies, we are talking about all the wheels of the energies of the body. You know very well what I mean: those famous chakras whose literal translation is not "centers" but "wheels"—because they are put to sacred tremoring and they keep whirling to infinity. You are the infinite!

STANZA 52

I venerate the spontaneous, tremoring, and wonderful
words of my master who had me cross the Ocean of
doubt.

May this jewel of knowledge lead all beings to reach
the true nature of reality, and may they keep this jewel
in the deepest part of their heart.

The Union of Joy and Emptiness

Tilopa is one of the Kashmiri siddhas who ensured the transmission of
Mahamudra by passing it on to his disciple Naropa, who in turn transmitted it to the ninth-century Tibetans. To this day, we can still see one
of his hermitages in the village of Tilokpur, near Dharmsala, in India.
Here is a song of his, as recounted by Chogyam Trungpa.

Homage to the Co-emergent Wisdom! *

Mahamudra cannot be shown;
But for you who are devoted to the guru, who have mastered
     the ascetic practices
And are forbearant in suffering, intelligent Naropa,
Take this to heart, my fortunate student.

Kye-ho! †

Look at the nature of this world,
Impermanent like a mirage or a dream;

---

*Note from cited text: Co-emergent Wisdom—the primordial wisdom, born simultane-
ously with ignorance, just as nirvana and samsara must come simultaneously into being.
†Note from cited text: Kye-ho!—Sanskrit: Hark! or Listen!

Even the mirage or dream does not exist.
Therefore, develop renunciation and abandon worldly
activities.

Renounce servants and kin, causes of passion and aggression.
Meditate alone in the forest, in retreats, in solitary places.
Remain in the state of nonmeditation.
If you attain nonattainment, then you have attained
mahamudra.

The dharma* of samsara is petty, causing passion and
aggression.
The things we have created have no substance; therefore, seek
the substance of the ultimate.
The dharma of mind cannot see the meaning of transcendent
mind.
The dharma of action cannot discover the meaning of
nonaction.

If you would attain the realization of transcendent mind and
nonaction,
Then cut the root of mind and let consciousness remain naked.
Let the polluted waters of mental activities clear.
Do not seek to stop projections, but let them come to rest of
themselves.
If there is no rejecting or accepting, then you are liberated in
the mahamudra.

When trees grow leaves and branches,
If you cut the roots, the many leaves and branches wither.
Likewise, if you cut the root of the mind,
The various mental activities will subside.

---

*Note from cited text: *dharma*—here taken as law, pattern, path.

The darkness that has collected in thousands of kalpas*
One torch will dispel.
Likewise, one moment's experience of luminous mind
Will dissolve the veil of karmic impurities.

Men of lesser intelligence who cannot grasp this,
Concentrate your awareness and focus on the breath.
Through different eye-gazes and concentration practices,
Discipline your mind until it rests naturally.

If you perceive space,
The fixed ideas of center and boundary dissolve.
Likewise, if mind perceives mind,
All mental activities will cease, you will remain in a state of
    nonthought.
And you will realize the supreme bodhi-citta.†
Vapors arising from the earth become clouds and then vanish
    into the sky;
It is not known where the clouds go when they have
    dissolved.
Likewise, the waves of thoughts derived from the mind
Dissolve when mind perceives mind.

Space has neither color nor shape;
It is changeless, it is not tinged by black or white.
Likewise, luminous mind has neither color nor shape;
It is not tinged by black or white, virtue or vice.

The sun's pure and brilliant essence
Cannot be dimmed by the darkness that endures for a
    thousand kalpas.

---

*Note from cited text: kalpas—Sanskrit: eons.
†Note from cited text: bodhi-citta—Sanskrit: awakened mind.

Likewise, the luminous essence of mind
Cannot be dimmed by the long kalpas of samsara.

Though it may be said that space is empty,
Space cannot be described.
Likewise, though it may be said that mind is luminous,
Naming it does not prove that it exists.
Space is completely without locality.
Likewise, mahamudra mind dwells nowhere.

Without change, rest loose in the primordial state;
There is no doubt that your bonds will loosen.
The essence of mind is like space;
Therefore, there is nothing which it does not encompass.

Let the movements of the body ease into genuineness,
Cease your idle chatter, let your speech become an echo,
Have no mind, but see the dharma of the leap.

The body, like a hollow bamboo, has no substance.
Mind is like the essence of space, having no place for
    thoughts.
Rest loose in your mind; neither hold it nor permit it to
    wander.
If mind has no aim, it is mahamudra.
Accomplishing this is the attainment of supreme
    enlightenment.

The nature of mind is luminous, without object of perception.
You will discover the path of the Buddha when there is no
    path of meditation.
By meditating on nonmeditation you will attain the supreme
    *bodhi.**

---

*Note from cited text: *bodhi*—Sanskrit: the awakened state.

This is the king of views—it transcends fixing and holding.*
This is the king of meditations—without wandering mind.
This is the king of actions—without effort.
When there is no hope and fear, you have realized the goal.

The unborn alaya† is without habits and veils.
Rest mind in the unborn essence; make no distinctions
   between meditation and post-meditation.
When projections exhaust the dharma of mind,
One attains the king of views, free from all limitations.

Boundless and deep is the supreme king of meditations.
Effortless self-existence is the supreme king of action.
Hopeless self-existence is the supreme king of the fruition.

In the beginning, mind is like a turbulent river.
In the middle, it is like the River Ganges, flowing slowly.
In the end, it is like the confluence of all rivers, like the
   meeting of son and mother.

The followers of Tantra, the Prajnaparamita,
The Vinaya,‡ the Sutras, and other religions—
All these, by their texts and philosophical dogmas,
Will not see the luminous mahamudra.

Having no mind, without desires,
Self-quieted, self-existing,

---

*Note from cited text: *fixing and holding—holding:* holding onto projections; *fixing:* believing in the existence of a projector.

†Note from cited text: unborn *alaya*—Sanskrit: the *dharmadhatu,* the primordial state beyond being and nonbeing.

‡Note from cited text: *Vinaya*—Sanskrit: the scriptures containing the hinayana rules of discipline.

It is like a wave of water.
Luminosity is veiled only by the rising of desire.

The real vow of samaya* *is broken by thinking in terms of*
precepts.
If you neither dwell, perceive, nor stray from the ultimate,
Then you are the holy practitioner, the torch which
illuminates darkness.
If you are without desire, if you do not dwell in extremes,
You will see the dharmas of all the teachings.

If you strive in this endeavor, you will free yourself from
samsaric imprisonment.
If you meditate in this way, you will burn the veil of karmic
impurities.
Therefore, you are known as "The Torch of the Doctrine."

Even ignorant people who are not devoted to this teaching
Could be saved by you from constantly drowning in the river
of samsara.

It is a pity that beings endure such suffering in the lower
realms.
Those who would free themselves from suffering should seek
a wise guru.
Being possessed by the adhishthana,† *one's mind will be freed.*

If you see seek a karma mudra,‡ *then the wisdom of the union*
of joy and emptiness will arise.

---

*Note from cited text: samaya—Sanskrit: the tantric vows of discipline.
†Note from cited text: adhishthana—Sanskrit: blessings, the atmosphere created by the guru.
‡Note from cited text: karma mudra—Sanskrit: one's consort in the practice of the third abhisheka, the third initiation.

The union of skillful means and knowledge brings blessings.
Bring it down and give rise to the mandala.
Deliver it to the places and distribute it throughout the body.

If there is no desire involved, then the union of joy and
emptiness will arise.
Gain long life, without white hairs, and you will wax like the
moon.
Become radiant, and your strength will be perfect.
Having speedily achieved the relative siddhis,* *one should*
seek the absolute siddhis.
May this pointed instruction in mahamudra remain in the
hearts of fortunate beings.[26]

---

*Note from cited text: *siddhis*—Sanskrit: miraculous powers.

Conclusion:
Should One Practice
Mahamudra?

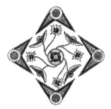

The tantrikas enter into a space without limits or reference points. They abandon all certainty and all concepts and apply the teaching in their contacts with the real, outside of all privileged frameworks.

The four essential points of the practice, which are sometimes jokingly called *sila*, or rules of conduct, are the following:

> Nonreality of phenomena, which leads to the perception that everything is real.
>
> Limitless spatiality, which leads to the perception that everything is consciousness and sacred tremor.
>
> Objectless solitude, which leads to the perception that solitude is merely a contraction of the absolute essence.
>
> Gracious spontaneity, which leads to the realization that everything is connected.

The practice of Mahamudra[1] is founded on four points:

The recognition of the absolute essence of the mind, which is identical and which unites all things.

The recognition of the creativity of the mind and of the fact that all emergence gushes like a spring from the absolute source and returns to it after a sensory, emotional, and mental circular journey.

The flow of consciousness being uninterrupted. When we lose our individual characteristics, we are in tune with totality.

The realization of the spacelike body. Sensory perceptions are space, emotions are space, mental perceptions are space.

To physical yoga we must add a yoga of the unending accompaniment of all emergences back to their source. This is perhaps the most important part of our work. It is founded on the perception that everything emerges from tranquillity and returns to it after a sensory, emotional, and mental journey. We learn, through the physical yoga of Tandava, Shiva's slow dance, to make the body more sensitive. An emotion is a sort of weather vane for changes in physical sensation. In automatic activity, these changes go unperceived. When the body has rediscovered its sensitivity, the slightest change is immediately noticed. From that moment on, the yogin becomes one with his emotion. He does not observe from a distant perspective; rather, he enters into the emotion as he would enter into the flow of a river that brings him back to the ocean of tranquillity. In our approach, we do not have the notion of a harmful or antagonistic emotion since all emotions, even the most violent, emerge from tranquillity only to return to tranquillity after a circular journey. Every blossoming brought back to its source leads us to tranquillity without leaving any unconscious baggage behind. Silence gradually appears, and unaddressed past emotions emerge in the present moment and are thus freed. There is no past emotion; everything happens in the immediate. The yogin gradually experiences great freedom. He no longer chooses; he allows himself to go with the flow of things. The fear of extreme states progressively disappears. No emergence is cut off or transformed. He seizes the raw matter of emotional reality.

After a few years of practice, we can taste an even deeper reality, which is truly the essence of Mahamudra: it is the realization that all emotion is free from the moment it emerges, and that its spatial nature is manifested throughout the course of the whole journey out and back. The transitory notion that an emotion leaves space and returns to it is naturally abandoned. The yogin then experiences each moment of the journey as spatial freedom.

The sign of having attained a deep level of yoga is the speed and the freedom with which the emergences circulate while silence is simultaneously experienced. This is the realization of Mahamudra. Suddenly, inner discourse is quieted. There is no longer prelude to action, commentary, or expectation. The body enters into continual sacred tremoring and reaches the limitless.

Tantric masters practicing Mahamudra teach consciousness, and it is very rare that they will substitute themselves for this consciousness in order to determine a life choice, a decision, an orientation. There is one very lovely exception:

One day, an old master who was on the verge of dying gave the transmission of the lineage to one of his disciples. The latter, taking advantage of the last moments with his master, could not help but make one last try:

"Master, when my disciples come to see me in the hope that I will give them instruction on a moral code in keeping with the teachings, is there really nothing to transmit to them?"

"Listen carefully," said the master in a last impulse of generosity. "What the mind loves is to form concepts, to compare, to put forth judgments, to get to the bottom of things, to form a fixed image of the teachings and transform them into certainties. Even though that is not really the view that we develop, give them permission to do this because they will not be able to help it. May they let their mind go wherever it likes, in total freedom, in absolute nonconformity, without being limited by injunctions and taboos. Try simply to get them to grasp that all movement is yoga from the moment when no one claims the propriety of this thought. Let thought go wherever it likes without getting to the point where you believe that it is your thought. Be like a light feather in a parade of the highest mountains: Carried by warm air currents, it rises; pushed by cold air currents it descends. It spins from left to right but does not believe that this movement issues from its own will."

"And what about sensory experiences?"

"What the eye likes above all is to contemplate harmonious forms and to let itself be carried by the joy of this vision. Let your eye embrace the forms that have an effect on it, explore the activity of matter and people, but do not go so far as to think that it is you who see the world. There is an immense arrogance in believing that our sight goes toward objects. Feel that the sky looks at you and that everything is sight."

"How should we consider the sense of touch?"

"What the skin likes above all is to be in contact with other skin, with delicate and living substances, to slip into running water, a lake, the ocean, or space. Therefore, let your skin go toward what attracts it and maintain the fundamental sacred tremor. Be like an instrument touched by the musician's body. Let all the harmonies that arise in you vibrate deeply, but try not to go so far that you imagine it is your skin that enters into contact with the universe."

"And for hearing?"

"What the ear likes above all is to hear melodious sounds, to taste the music of people and of world. Free your hearing from all limitation, and allow it to taste harmony, but do not go so far that you think it is your hearing that listens to the universe."

"For taste?"

"What the tongue likes above all is to be in contact with delicious flavors, to explore the world, its sources and cavities, its dews and its saps. Let your mouth go toward reality, but do not go so far that you believe it is your mouth that embraces the world."

"And for smell?"

"What the nose likes is to be in contact with delicious fragrances. It likes to taste the delicious scents of plants and people, it likes to breathe space, the rain that falls on a forest, the delicious smell of a person who abandons himself. Therefore, allow your nose to breathe in the world, but do not go so far that you believe it is your nose."

"What happens if the yogin and the yogini succeed in this marvel?"

"Then all perception is spatial perception, and all the beauty of the world brings us back unceasingly to the unlimited. But if the ego collects our sensory impressions, it uses them to build a fortress and isolate itself from the world. Taking pleasure in beauty is the most profound yoga if no one captures the perception. This is my last teaching, it is the accomplishment of the whole Mahamudra approach. Pass it on to those who are worthy of it and who will be able to remain above the senses like the sun and moon remain above the clouds."

Then the old master left, he looked at the valley one last time, breathed in the smell of the forest, caressed a rock, sat upon the ground, drank a drop of dew off a leaf, and passed on, abandoning his body, his emotions, and his thought to space. [2]

Padmasambhava revealed the secret of the ultimate practice, such as he had revealed it to his consort, Yeshé Tsogyal, princess of Karchen:

Place your sight in space, straight in front of you, without moving the eyeballs, relax your awareness so that it will be sharp/keen, luminous, awakened, and embracing totality. May it be free from the fixation of observer and observed. [3]

Although there are many profound key points in the body, rest free and relaxed, as you feel comfortable. Everything is included in simply that.

Although there are many key points on speech such as breath control and mantra recitation, stop speaking and rest like a mute. Everything is included in simply that.

Although there are many key points of mind such as concentrating, relaxing, projecting, dissolving, and focusing inward, everything is included in simply letting it rest in its natural state, free and easy, without fabrication. . . .

1. View as a mere convention that the root of all phenomena is contained within your own bodhicitta awareness, the primordial purity of nonarising.

2. See that this bodhicitta awareness is primordially enlightened since it does not possess any constructs such as a watcher or an object to be watched.

3. Recognize that whatever thoughts or fixations arise within, the state of this awareness is primordially empty and luminous awareness itself.

4. Recognize that whatever outer appearances may arise do not possess any identity whatsoever from the very moment they are experienced, and therefore do not transcend being the display of dharmata.

5. Experience the nonduality of objects and mind as the innate great bliss, free from accepting and rejecting, affirming or denying.

   In particular, experience all the disturbing emotions and suffering as the sacred path of enlightenment.

6. Realize that sentient beings, from the moment they are experienced, do not possess any true existence and therefore that samsara is the primordial purity of nonarising and does not have to be abandoned.

7. Realize that everything experienced as kayas and wisdoms is contained within your mind and therefore that buddhahood is beyond being accomplished.

8. Do this and you will be the successor of glorious Samanthabhadra.*[4]

---

*Samantha means "extending through space," and Bhadra means "Great Virtue." This Bodhisatva rides on an elephant with six tusks (the six senses).

Vijnanabhairava Tantra

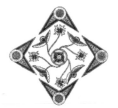

The *Vijnanabhairava Tantra,* a text written by the Shaivite School of Kashmir around the first century A.D., represents "the quintessence of all the tantras." It stands first and foremost on the plane of absolute reality, where it touches the deepest roots of the spirit. This "tantra of supreme consciousness" is probably the most extraordinary sum total of yogic methods ever brought together. It offers an extremely original approach that utilizes the complete spectrum of thought, emotion, and sensation as a mystical path. Far from impelling the devotee to renounce the world, on the contrary, it urges him or her to touch the world so profoundly that he or she discovers the absolute at the very heart of reality.

Starting with the opening stanzas (7 to 17) Shiva places the practice outside ritual form in order to establish it "in the fullness of the aware-ness of the Self." It simply involves rediscovering our divine essence of

"Shiva/Shakti" through the practice of exercises that focus our attention, allowing us to see that the divine is at the very heart of the awareness of breath, sensations, emotions, and thoughts.

The great originality of this tantra resides in the fact that it rehabilitates negative and disturbing emotions into great yogic paths. In this way, jealousy, fear, violence, anguish, and projection are valorized as moments of the complete oneness of the personality that can provide access to cosmic consciousness. The tantrika rejects no facet of human experience but seeks only to use reality as a door that provides access to higher mystical states. Reality and illusion thus find themselves combined in this quest that defies duality. For the tantrika, there is nothing that may not be the path.

Bhairava and Bhairavi, lovingly united in the same knowledge, left the undifferentiated state so their dialog may enlighten all beings.

1. Bhairava's Shakti, Bhairavi, said:
O God, who manifests the universe and makes light of this manifestation, you are none else than my Self. I have received the teachings of the Trika, which is the quintessence of all the scriptures. However, I still have some doubts.

2–4. O God, from the standpoint of absolute reality, what is the essential nature of Bhairava? Does it reside in the energy of the phonemes? In the realization of Bhairava's essential nature? In a particular mantra? In the three Shakti? In the presence of the mantra that lives in every word? In the power of the mantra present in each particle of the universe? Does it reside in the chakras? In the sound Ha? Or is it only the Shakti?

5–6. That which is composed, is it born out of both immanent and transcendent energy, or only out of immanent energy? If it were the product of transcendent energy only, then transcendence itself would have no object. Transcendence cannot be differentiated in sounds and particles for its undivided nature cannot be expressed in the many.

7–10. O Lord, may your grace do away with my doubts! Excellent! Your questions, O Beloved, are the essence of the Tantras. I will reveal to you a secret teaching. All that is perceived as a composed form of the sphere of Bhairava must be considered as phantasmagoria, magical illusion, a ghost city hanging in the sky. Such a description only aims to drive those who fall prey to illusion and mundane activity toward contemplation. Such teachings are meant for those who are interested in rituals and external practices and stuck in duality.

11–13. From an absolute standpoint, Bhairava is not associated with letters, nor with phonemes, nor with the three Shakti, nor with breaking through the chakras, nor with any other belief, and Shakti does not constitute his essence. All these concepts taught in the scriptures are aimed at those whose mind is still too immature to grasp the supreme reality. They are mere appetizers meant to spur aspirants toward ethical behavior and spiritual practice so that they can realize someday that the ultimate nature of Bhairava is not separate from their own Self.

14–17. Mystical ecstasy isn't subject to dualistic thought, it is completely free from any notion of location, space, or time. This truth can only be touched by experience. It can only be reached by those entirely freed from duality and ego, and firmly, fully established in the consciousness of the Self. This state of Bhairava is filled with the pure bliss of unity between tantrika and the universe. Only this state is the Shakti. In the reality of one's own nature thus recognized, containing the entire universe, one reaches the highest sphere. Who then could be worshipped? Who then could be fulfilled by this worship? Only this condition recognized as supreme is the great Goddess.

18–19. Since there is no difference between the Shakti and the one who embodies her, nor between substance and object, the Shakti is identical to the Self. The energy of the flames is nothing but the fire. All distinction is but a prelude to the path of true knowledge.

20–21. The one who reaches the Shakti grasps the nondistinction between Shiva and Shakti and enters the door to the divine. As space is recognized when illuminated by sun rays, so Shiva is recognized through the energy of Shakti, which is the essence of the Self.

22–23. O supreme God! You who bears a trident and a garland of skulls, how to reach the absolute plenitude of the Shakti that transcends all notions, all descriptions and abolishes time and space? How to realize this nonseparation from the universe? In what sense is it said that the supreme Shakti is the secret door to the state of Bhairava? Can you answer in common language these absolute questions?

24. The supreme Shakti reveals herself when inbreath and outbreath are born and die at the two extreme points, top and bottom. Thus, between two breaths, experience infinite space.

25. Between inbreath and outbreath, between stopping and going, when breath stands still at the two extreme points, inner heart and outer heart, two empty spaces will be revealed to you: Bhairava and Bhairavi.

26. With a relaxed body when exhaling and inhaling, lose your mind and perceive your heart, the energy center where the absolute essence of Bhairava flows.

27. When you have breathed in or out completely, when the breath movement stops on its own, in this universal lull, the thought of *me* disappears and the Shakti reveals herself.

28. Consider the Shakti as bright, subtler and subtler light, carried upward through the lotus stem, from center to center, by the energy of the breath. When it subsides in the upper center, it is Bhairava's awakening.

29. The heart opens up and, from center to center, Kundalini rushes up like lightning. Then Bhairava's glory is manifested.

30. Meditate on the twelve energy centers, the twelve related letters and free yourself from materiality to reach the supreme subtlety of Shiva.

31. Focus your attention between your eyebrows, keep your mind free from any dualistic thought, let your form be filled with breath essence up to the top of your head, and there, soak in radiant spatiality.

32. Imagine the five colored circles of a peacock feather to be your five senses disseminated in unlimited space and reside in the spatiality of your own heart.

33. Void, wall, whatever the object of contemplation, it is the matrix of the spatiality of your own mind.

34. Close your eyes, see the whole space as if it were absorbed in your own head, direct your gaze inwards, and there, see the spatiality of your true nature.

35. The inner channel is the Goddess, like a lotus stem, red inside, blue outside. It runs across your body. Meditating on its internal vacuity, you will reach divine spatiality.

36. Plug the seven openings of your head with your fingers and merge into the bindu, the infinite space between your eyebrows.

37. If you meditate in your heart, in the upper center or between your eyes, the spark which will dissolve discursive thought will ignite, like when brushing eyelids with fingers. You will then melt into supreme consciousness.

38. Enter the center of spontaneous sound that resonates on its own like the uninterrupted sound of a waterfall. Or, sticking your fingers in your ears, hear the sound of sounds and reach Brahman, the immensity.

39. O Bhairavi, sing OM, the mantra of the love union of Shiva and Shakti, slowly and consciously. Enter the sound and when it fades away, slip into freedom of being.

40. Focus on the emergence or the disappearance of a sound, then reach the ineffable plenitude of the void.

41. By being totally present to song, to music, enter spatiality with each sound that rises and dissolves into it.

42. Visualize a letter, let yourself be filled by its radiance. With open awareness, enter first the sonority of the letter, then a subtler and subtler sensation. When the letter dissolves into space, be free.

43. When you contemplate the luminous spatiality of your own body radiating in every direction, you free yourself from duality and you merge into space.

44. If you contemplate simultaneously spatiality above and at the base, then bodiless energy will carry you beyond dualistic thought.

45. Reside simultaneously in the spatiality at the base, in your heart, and above your head. Thus, in the absence of dualistic thought, divine consciousness blossoms.

46. In one moment, perceive nonduality in one spot of your body, penetrate this limitless space and reach the essence freed from duality.

47. O gazelle-eyed one, let ether pervade your body, merge in the indescribable spatiality of your own mind.

48. Suppose your body to be pure radiant spatiality contained by your skin and reach the limitless.

49. O beauty! Senses disseminated in your heart space, perceive the essence of the Shakti as indescribably fine gold powder that glitters in your heart and from there pours into space. Then you will know supreme bliss.

50. When your body is pervaded with consciousness, your one-pointed mind dissolves into your heart and you penetrate reality.

51. Fix your mind in your heart when engaged in worldly activity, thus agitation will disappear and in a few days the indescribable will happen.

52. Focus on a fire, fierier and fierier, which raises from your feet and burns you entirely. When there is nothing left but ashes scattered by the wind, know the tranquillity of space that returns to space.

53. See the entire world as a blazing inferno. Then, when all has turned into ashes, enter bliss.

54. If subtler and subtler tattvas are absorbed into their own origin, the supreme Goddess will be revealed to you.

55. Reach an intangible breath focused between your eyes, then when the light appears let the Shakti come down to your heart and there, in the radiant presence, at the moment of sleep, attain the mastery of dreams and know the mystery of death itself.

56. Consider the entire universe to be dissolving in subtler and subtler forms until it merges into pure consciousness.

57. If, boundless in space, you meditate on Shiva tattva, which is the quintessence of the entire universe, you will know ultimate ecstasy.

58. O great Goddess, perceive the spatiality of the universe, and become the jar that contains it.

59. Look at a bowl or a container without seeing its sides or the matter that composes it. In little time become aware of space.

60. Abide in an infinitely spacious place, devoid of trees, hills, dwellings. Let your gaze dissolve in empty space, until your mind relaxes.

61. In the empty space that separates two instants of awareness, radiant spatiality is revealed.

62. Just as you get the impulse to do something, stop. Then, being no more in the preceding impulse nor in the following one, realization blossoms intensely.

63. Contemplate over the undivided forms of your own body and those of the entire universe as being of an identical nature. Thus will your omnipresent being and your own form rest in unity and you will reach the very nature of consciousness.

64. In any activity, concentrate on the gap between inbreath and outbreath. Thus attain to bliss.

65. Feel your substance: bone, flesh, and blood, saturated with cosmic essence, and know supreme bliss.

66. O gazelle-eyed beauty, consider the winds to be your own body of bliss. When you quiver, reach the luminous presence.

67. When your senses shiver and your mind becomes still, enter the energy of breath, and, when you feel pins and needles, know supreme joy.

68. When you practice a sex ritual, let thought reside in the quivering of your senses like wind in the leaves, and reach the celestial bliss of ecstatic love.

69. At the start of the union, be in the fire of the energy released by intimate sensual pleasure. Merge into the divine Shakti and keep burning in space, avoiding the ashes at the end. These delights are in truth those of the Self.

70. O Goddess! The sensual pleasure of the intimate bliss of union can be reproduced at any moment by the radiant presence of the mind that remembers intensely this pleasure.

71. When you meet again with a loved one, be in this bliss totally and penetrate the luminous space.

72. At the time of euphoria and expansion caused by delicate foods and drinks, be total in this delight and, through it, taste supreme bliss.

73. Merge in the joy felt at the time of musical pleasure or pleasure from other senses. If you immerse in this joy, you reach the divine.

74. Wherever you find satisfaction, the very essence of bliss will be revealed to you if you remain in this place without mental wavering.

75. At the point of sleep, when sleep has not yet come and wakefulness vanishes, at this very point, know the supreme Goddess.

76. In summer, when your gaze dissolves in the endlessly clear sky, penetrate this light that is the essence of your own mind.

77. You will enter the spatiality of your own mind at the moment when intuition frees itself through steadiness of gaze, love uninterrupted, sucking, violent feelings, agony, or death.

78. Comfortably seated, feet and hands unsupported, enter the space of ineffable fullness.

79. In a comfortable position, hands open at shoulder level, an area of radiant spatiality gradually pervades the armpits, ravishes the heart, and brings about profound peace.

80. Steadily gazing without blinking at a pebble, a piece of wood, or any other ordinary object, thought loses all props and rapidly attains to Shiva/Shakti.

81. Open your mouth, place your mind in your tongue at the center of the oral cavity, exhale with the sound HA and know a peaceful presence to the world.

82. Laying flat, see your body as supportless. Let your thought dissolve into space, and then the contents of the inner core consciousness will dissolve too, and you will experience pure presence, freed from dreams.

83. O Goddess, enjoy the extremely slow movements of your body, of a mount, of a vehicle and, with peace in mind, sink into divine spirit.

84. Gaze at a very clear sky without blinking. Tensions dissolve along with your gaze and then reach the awesome steadiness of Bhairava.

85. Enter the radiant spatiality of Bhairava scattered in your own head, leave space and time, be Bhairava.

86. When you reach Bhairava by dissolving duality when awake, when this spatial presence continues into dream, and when you then cross the night of deep sleep as the very form of Bhairava, know the infinite splendor of awake consciousness.

87. During a dark and moonless night, eyes open in the dark, let your whole being melt into this obscurity and attain to the form of Bhairava.

88. Eyes closed, dissolve into darkness, then open your eyes and identify with the awesome form of Bhairava.

89. When an obstacle gets in the way of gratification through senses, seize this instant of spatial emptiness, which is the very essence of meditation.

90. With all your being, utter a word ending in "AH" and in the "H" let yourself be swept away by the gushing flow of wisdom.

91. When you focus your structure-free mind on the final sound of a letter, immensity is revealed.

92. Waking, sleeping, dreaming, consciousness free from any prop, know yourself as radiant spatial presence.

93. Pierce a place on your body and, through this one spot, attain to the radiant domain of Bhairava.

94. When through contemplation, ego, active intellect, and mind are revealed as empty, any form becomes a limitless space and the very root of duality dissolves.

95. Illusion perturbs, the five sheaths obstruct vision, separations imposed by dualistic thought are artificial.

96. When you become aware of a desire, consider it the time of a snap of fingers, then suddenly let go. Then it returns to the space it just came out of.

97. Before desiring, before knowing: Who am I, where am I? such is the true nature of I, such is the spatial depth of reality.

98. When desire or knowledge have manifested, forget their object and focus your mind on objectless desire or knowledge as being the Self. Then you will reach deep reality.

99. Any particular knowledge is deceptive. When thirst for knowledge arises, immediately realize the spatiality of knowledge itself and be Shiva/Shakti.

100. Consciousness is everywhere, there is no differentiation. Realize this deeply and thus triumph over time.

101. In a state of extreme desire, anger, greed, confusion, pride, or envy, enter your own heart and discover the underlying peace.

102. If you perceive the entire universe as phantasmagoria, an ineffable joy will arise in you.

103. O Bhairavi, do not reside in pleasure nor in pain, instead be constantly in the ineffable spatial reality that links them.

104. When you realize that you are in every thing, the attachment to body dissolves, joy and bliss arise.

105. Desire exists in you as in every thing. Realize that it also resides in objects and in all that the mind can grasp. Then, discovering the universality of desire, enter its radiant space.

106. Every living being perceives subject and object, but the tantrika resides in their union.

107. Feel the consciousness of each being as your own.

108. Free the mind of all props and attain to nonduality. Then, gazelle-eyed one, limited self becomes absolute Self.

109. Shiva is omnipresent, omnipotent, and omniscient. Since you have the attributes of Shiva, you are similar to him. Recognize the divine in yourself.

110. Waves are born of the ocean and get lost in it, flames arise and die, the sun shows.

111. Wander or dance to exhaustion in utter spontaneity. Then, suddenly, drop to the ground and in this fall be total. There absolute essence is revealed.

112. Suppose you are gradually deprived of energy and knowledge. At the moment of this dissolution, your true being will be revealed.

113. O Goddess, hear the ultimate mystical teaching: you need only fix your gaze onto space without blinking to attain to the spatiality of your own mind.

114. Stop sound perception by plugging your ears. Contracting the anus, start resonating and touch that which is not subject to space or time.

115. At the edge of a well, gaze motionless into its depths until wonder seizes you and merge into space.

116. When your mind wanders externally or internally, it is then precisely that the shaivist state manifests. Where could thought take refuge to not savor this state?

117. Spirit is in you and all around you. When all is pure spatial consciousness, attain the essence of plenitude.

118. In stupor, anxiety, extreme feelings, at the edge of a precipice, running from the battlefield, in hunger or terror, or even when you sneeze, the essence of the spatiality of your own mind can be seized.

119. When the sight of a certain place brings back memories, let your mind relive these instants; then, when memories fade away, one step further, know omnipresence.

120. Look at an object, then slowly withdraw your eyes. Then withdraw your thoughts and become the receptacle of ineffable plenitude.

121. The intuition that springs from the intensity of passionate devotion flows into space, frees you and lets you attain to the domain of Shiva/Shakti.

122. Attention focused on a single object, you penetrate any object. Relax then in the spatial plenitude of your own Self.

123. Purity praised by ignorant religious people seems impure to the tantrika. Free yourself from dualistic thought, and do not consider anything as pure or impure.

124. Understand that the spatial reality of Bhairava is present in every thing, in every being, and be this reality.

125. Happiness resides in equality between extreme feelings. Reside in your own heart and attain to plenitude.

126. Free yourself from hatred as well as from attachment. Then, knowing neither aversion nor bond, slip into the divine inside your own heart.

127. Open and sweet-hearted one, meditate on what cannot be known, what cannot be grasped. All duality being out of reach, where could consciousness settle to escape from ecstasy?

128. Contemplate empty space, attain to nonperception, nondistinction, the elusive, beyond being and not-being: reach nonspace.

129. When thought is drawn to an object, utilize this energy. Go beyond the object, and there, fix your thought on this empty and luminous space.

130. Bhairava is one with your radiant consciousness; singing the name of Bhairava, one becomes Shiva.

131. When you state: "I exist," "I think this or that," "such thing belongs to me," touch that which is unfounded and beyond such statements, know the limitless and find peace.

132. "Eternal, omnipotent, supportless, Goddess of the whole manifested world . . . " Be that one and attain to Shiva/Shakti.

133. What you call universe is an illusion, a magical appearance. To be happy, consider it as such.

134. Without dualistic thought, what could limit consciousness?

135. In reality, bond and liberation exist only for those who are terrified by the world and ignore their fundamental nature: the universe is reflected in the mind like the sun on the waters.

136. At the moment where your attention awakens through sensory organs, enter the spatiality of your own heart.

137. When knower and known are one and the same, the Self shines brightly.

138. O beloved, when mind, intellect, energy, and limited self vanish, then appears the wonderful Bhairava.

139. O Goddess, I just taught you one hundred and twelve dharana. One who knows them escapes from dualistic thought and attains to perfect knowledge.

140. One who realizes one single of these dharana becomes Bhairava himself. His word gets enacted and he obtains the power to transmit the Shakti at will.

141–144. O Goddess, the being who masters one single of these practices frees himself from old age and death, he acquires supernormal powers, all yogini and yogin cherish him and he presides over their secret meetings. Liberated in the very middle of activity and reality, he is free.

The Goddess said:
O Lord, let us follow this wonderful reality that is the nature of the supreme Shakti! Who then is worshipped? Who is the worshipper? Who enters contemplation? Who is contemplated? Who gives the oblation and who receives it? What gets sacrificed and to whom? O gazelle-eyed one, all these practices are those of the external path. They fit gross aspirations.

145. Only the contemplation of the highest reality is the practice of the tantrika. What resonates spontaneously in oneself is the mystical formula.

146. A stable and characterless mind, there is true contemplation. Colorful visualizations of divinities are nothing but artifice.

147. Worship does not consist in offerings but in the realization that the heart is supreme consciousness, free from dualistic thought. In perfect ardor, Shiva/Shakti dissolve in the Self.

148. If one penetrates one single element of the yoga described here, one will know a plenitude spreading from day to day to reach the highest perfection.

149. When one casts into the fire of supreme reality the five elements, the senses and their objects, the dualistic mind and even vacuity, then there is true offering to the Gods.

150–151. O supreme Goddess, here the sacrifice is nothing else than spiritual satisfaction characterized by bliss. The real pilgrimage, O Pārvati, is the absorption in the Shakti, which destroys all stains and protects all beings. How could there be another kind of worship and who would be worshipped?

152. The essence of the Self is universal. It is autonomy, bliss, and consciousness. Absorption in this essence is the ritual bath.

153. Offerings, devotee, supreme Shakti are but one. This is supreme devotion.

154. Breath comes out, breath comes in, sinuous in itself. Perfectly tuned to the breath, Kundalini, the great Goddess, rises up. Transcendent and immanent, she is the highest place of pilgrimage.

155. Thus, deeply established in the rite of the great bliss, fully present to the rise of divine energy, thanks to the Goddess, the yogin will attain to supreme Bhairava.

155a–156. Air is exhaled with the sound SA and inhaled with the sound HAM. Then reciting of the mantra HAMSA is continuous. Breath is the mantra, repeated twenty-one thousand times, day and night. It is the mantra of the great Goddess.

157–160. O Goddess! I just gave you the ultimate, unsurpassed mystical teachings. Let them only be taught to generous beings, to those who revere the Masters' lineage, to the intuitive minds freed from cognitive wavering and doubt, and to those who will practice them. For without practice, transmission gets diluted, and those who had the wonderful opportunity to receive these teachings return to suffering and illusion even though they have held an eternal treasure in their hands. O God, I have now grasped the heart of the teachings and the quintessence of Tantra. This life will have to be left behind, but why renounce the heart of the Shakti? As space is recognized when lit by sunrays, so is Shiva told through the energy of Shakti, which is the essence of the Self.

Then, Shiva and Shakti, glowing in bliss, merged again in the undifferentiated.[1]

APPENDIX 2

The Natural Liberation through Naked Vision, Identifying Intelligence

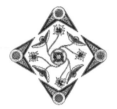

The following is an alternate translation of the song by Padmasambhava that is presented at the end of the commentary on the second flow. The reader can find this translation in *Essential Tibetan Buddhism*, by Robert A. F. Thurman.[1]

> *EMA HOH!*
> *The one mind that pervades all life and liberation*
> *Though it is the primal nature, it is not recognized,*
> *Though its brilliant intelligence is uninterrupted, it is not*
>   *faced,*
> *Though it ceaselessly arises everywhere, it is not recognized.*
> *To make known just this objective nature,*

The three-times victors proclaimed the inconceivable
Eighty-four thousand Dharma teachings,
Teaching none other than this realization.
Though Scriptures are measureless as the sky,
Their importance is three words identifying intelligence.
This direct introduction to the intention of the Victors—
Just this is the entry into freedom from progression.

KYAI HO! [Victory!]
Fortunate children! Listen here!
"Mind"—though this great word is so well known—
People do not know it, know it wrongly or only partially;
And by their not understanding its reality precisely,
They come up with inconceivable philosophical claims.
The common, alienated individual, not realizing this,
By not understanding her nature on her own,
Suffers roaming through six life forms in three realms.
Such is the fault of not realizing this reality of the mind.

Disciples and hermit Buddhas claim realization
Of a partial selflessness but do not know this exactly.
Bound up in claims from their treatises and theories,
They do not behold clear light transparency.

Disciples and hermits are shut out by clinging to subject and
*   object,*
Centrists are shut out by extremism about the two realities,
Ritual and performance Tantrists, by extremism in service and
*   practice,*
And great (Maha) and pervasive (Anu) Tantrists,
By clinging to the duality of realm and intelligence.
They err by remaining dualistic in nonduality,
By not communing nondually, they do not awaken.
All life and liberation inseparable from their own minds,

They still roam the life-cycle on vehicles of quitting and
* choosing.*

Therefore, absorbing all created things in your free inaction,
Realize the great natural liberation of all things from this
* teaching*
Of natural liberation through naked seeing of your own
* intelligence!*
Thus in the great perfection, everything is perfect . . .

"Mind," this bright process of intelligence,
In one way exists and in another way does not.
It is origin of pleasure and pain of life and liberation.
It is accepted as essential to the eleven vehicles of liberation.

Its names are countless in various contexts.
Some call this mind "the mind-reality."
Some fundamentalists call it "self."
Some disciples call it "selflessness."
Idealists call it by the name of "mind."
Some call it "Transcendental Wisdom."
Some call it "the Buddha nature."
Some call it "the Great Seal."
Some call it "the Soul Drop."
Some call it "the Truth Realm."
Some call it "the Foundation."
Some call it "the Ordinary."

To introduce the three-point entrance to this itself—
Realize past awareness as trackless, clear, and void,
Future awareness as unproduced and new,
And present awareness as staying natural, uncontrived.

Thus knowing time in its very ordinary way,
When you nakedly yourself regard yourself,
Your looking is transparent, nothing to be seen.
This is naked, immediate, clear intelligence.

It is clear voidness with nothing established,
Purity of clarity-voidness-nonduality;
Not permanent, free of any intrinsic status,
Not annihilated, bright and distinct,
Not unity, multidiscerning clarity,
Without plurality, indivisible, one in taste,
Nor derivative, self-aware, it is this very reality.

This objective introduction to the actuality of things
Contains complete in one the indivisible three bodies.
The Truth Body, the voidness free of intrinsic status,
The Beatific Body, bright with freedom's natural energy,
The Emanation Body, ceaselessly arising everywhere—
The reality is these three complete in one.

To introduce the forceful method to enter this very reality,
Your own awareness right now is just this!
In being just this uncontrived natural clarity,
Why do you say, "I don't understand the nature of the mind"?
As here there is nothing to meditate upon,
In just this uninterrupted clarity intelligence,
Why do you say, "I don't see the actuality of the mind"?
Since the thinker in the mind is just it,
Why do you say, "Even searching I can't find it"?
Since here there is nothing to be done,
Why do you say, "Whatever I do, it doesn't succeed"?
As it is sufficient to stay put uncontrived,
Why do you say, "I can't stay still"?
As it is all right to be content with inaction,

Why do you say, "I am not able to do it"?
Since clear, aware, and void are automatically indivisible,
Why do you say, "Practice is not effective"?
Since it is natural, spontaneous, free of cause and condition,
Why do you say, "Seeking, it cannot be found"?
Since thought and natural liberation are simultaneous,
Why do you say, "Remedies are impotent"?
Since your very intelligence is just this,
Why do you say, "I do not know this"?

Be sure mind's nature is groundless voidness;
Your mind is insubstantial like empty space—
Like it or not, look at your own mind!
Not fastening to the view of annihilative voidness,
Be sure spontaneous wisdom has always been clear,
Spontaneous in itself like the essence of the sun—
Like it or not, look at your own mind!

Be sure that intelligent wisdom is uninterrupted,
Like a continuous current of a river—
Like it or not, look at your own mind!
Be sure it will not be known by thinking various reasons,
Its movement insubstantial like breezes in the sky—
Like it or not, look at your own mind!
Be sure that what appears is your own perception;
Appearance is natural perception, like a reflection in a
  mirror—
Like it or not, look at your own mind!
Be sure that all signs are liberated on the spot,
Self-originated, self-delivered, like clouds in the sky—
Like it or not, look at your own mind!

Vision-voidness natural liberation
Is brilliant void Body of Truth.

Realizing Buddhahood is not achieved by paths—
Vajrasattva is beheld right now. . . .

Therefore, to see intuitively your own naked intelligence,
This Natural Liberation through Naked Vision *is extremely*
    deep.
So investigate this reality of your own intelligence.

Profound! Sealed!

EMA!

Notes

Preface

1. In Daniel Odier, *Tantra Yoga, le tantra de la connaissance suprême* (Paris: Albin Michel, 1998 and 2004). There is an English translation of the root text on the author's Web site: www.danielodier.com.
2. Kalu Rinpoché, in *La Voie du Bouddha selon la tradition tibetaine*, texts assembled and translated by the Lama Denis Teundroup (Seuil: Points Sagesse, 1993). English translation here by Clare Frock.
3. Guilaine Mala in *Tch'an, Zen, racines et floraisons,* ed., Lilian Silburn. Hermès New Series 4. (Paris: Les Deux Océans, 1985), 387–424.
4. Takpo Tashi Namgyal, foreword by Chögyam Trungpa, *Mahamudra: The Quintessence of Mind and Meditation* (Delhi: Motilal Banarsidass, 1993).
5. Karma Chagmé, *A Spacious Path to Freedom: Practical Instructions on the Union of Mahamudra and Atiyoga,* trans., B. Alan Wallace (Ithaca, N.Y.: Snow Lion Publications, 1998).
6. *Bodhidharma,* treatise by Bodhidharma translated from the Chinese by Faure (Seuil: Points Sagesse, 1993).
7. See *The Secret Teachings of the Nyingmapa* 9 (Ithaca, N.Y.: Snow Lion Publications), and Teundroup, *La Voie du Bouddha.*
8. Alain Daniélou, *Shiva et Dyonisos* (Paris: Le Rocher), 1985.
9. Herbert Guenther, *Ecstatic Spontaneity: Saraha's Three Cycles of Doha* (Berkeley, Calif.: Asian Humanities Press, 1993), 135–137, stanzas 41 and 45.
10. See www.zhaozhou-chan.com

The Tantric Song of the Sacred Tremor

1. For more on the sacred tremor, see also Daniel Odier, *Desire: The Tantric Path to Awakening* (Rochester, Vt.: Inner Traditions International, 2001).

2. First translated into French by the author, from Lalita Devi's unpublished English version. *Translator's note*: The English version presented here has been translated from the author's written French, with his guidance and approval.

First Flow (Stanzas 1–16)

1. Savari, in Takpo Tashi Namgyal, *Mahamudra: The Quintessence of Mind and Meditation,* ed. and trans., Lobsang P. Lhalungpa. (Boston: Shambhala, 1986), 317, section 298 F.
2. Ibid., section 298 B.
3. English translation of the French from the author's notebooks by Clare Frock. Original source is most likely Namgyal, *Mahamudra.* Both author and translator were unable to locate this passage.
4. Namgyal, *Mahamudra,* 281, section 266 B.
5. Ibid., 322, section 303 F.
6. Ibid., 324, section 305 F.
7. Ibid., 325, section 305 B.
8. Ibid., 326, section 306 F.
9. Ibid., 327–328, sections 306 B and 307 F.
10. From "Song of Enlightenment" by Yung Chia Hsuan Chueh, in Master Sheng-yen, trans./ed., *The Poetry of Enlightenment: Poems by Ancient Ch'an Masters* (Elmhurst, N.Y.: Dharma Drum Publications, 1987), 49.
11. Abhinavagupta, in Daniel Odier, *Tantra: Spontanéité de l'extase* (Paris: Actes Sud, 2000). English translation by Clare Frock.
12. Mala, *Tch'an, Zen, racines et floraisons.* English translation here by Clare Frock.
13. Ibid. English translation here by Clare Frock.
14. Namgyal, *Mahamudra,* 334–335, sections 313 B–313 F.
15. Jerome Edou, *Machig Labdrön and the Foundations of Chod* (Ithaca, N.Y.: Snow Lion Publications, 1996), 165–170.

Second Flow (Stanzas 17–27)

1. J. C. Cleary and Thomas Cleary, trans./eds., *Zen Letters: Teachings of Yuanwu* (Boston: Shambhala, 1994), 55.
2. Thomas Cleary, trans./ed., *Zen Essence: The Science of Freedom* (Boston: Shambhala, 1989), 53.
3. English translation of the French from the author's notebooks by Clare Frock.
4. Constantin R. Bailly, *Shaiva Devotional Songs of Kashmir: A Translation and Study of Utpaladeva's Shivastotravali* (Albany, N.Y.: SUNY Press, 1987), 32–33. From The First Song, "The Pleasure of Devotion," stanzas 21 and 25.

5. Foyan, *Instant Zen: Waking up in the Present*. Trans., Thomas Cleary. (Berkeley, Calif.: North Atlantic Books, 1994), 91.

6. Author and translator were unable to locate this passage. English translation of the French from the author's notebooks by Clare Frock.

7. Foyan, *Instant Zen*, 27, and Cleary, *Zen Essence*, 42.

8. Author and translator were unable to locate this passage. English translation of the French from the author's notebooks by Clare Frock.

9. Foyan, *Instant Zen*, 8.

10. Ibid., 7.

11. Guenther, *Ecstatic Spontaneity: Saraha's Three Cycles of Doha*, 135–137, stanzas 40, 41, and 45.

12. *Tch'an, Zen, racines et floraisons*, English translation here by Clare Frock.

13. Daniel Odier, trans., *Lalla, Chants mystiques du tantrisme cachemirien* (Seuil: Points Sagesse, 2001). English translation here by Clare Frock.

14. *Le Secret de la déesse Tripura*. Translated by Serge Hulin (Paris: Éditions Fayard, 1985). English translation here by Clare Frock. There is an English translation as well by Swami Sri Ramananda Saraswati, in *Tripura Rahasya: The Secret of the Supreme Goddess* (Bloomington, Ind.: World Wisdom, 2002).

15. John Myrdhin Reynolds, *Self-Liberation through Seeing with Naked Awareness* (Ithaca, N.Y.: Snow Lion Publications, 2000), 9–28. For another translation, see Appendix 2, "Natural Liberation Through Naked Vision, Identifying Intelligence," translated by Robert A. F. Thurman.

Third Flow (Stanzas 28–52)

1. English translation of the French from the author's notebooks by Clare Frock.

2. *Huang Po, Maître Tch'an du IXème siècle*. Entretiens, Présentation et traduction du chinois by Patrick Carré (Seuil: Points Sagesse, 1993). English translation here by Clare Frock.

3. *Tch'an, Zen, racines et floraisons*. English translation here by Clare Frock.

4. English translation of the French from the author's notebooks by Clare Frock.

5. Mazu, *Les entretiens de Mazu*. Introduction by Catherine Despeux (Paris: Les Deux Océans, 1989). English translation here by Clare Frock. There is also an English edition of this book: *Sun Face Buddha: The Teachings of Ma-tsu and Ung-chou School of Ch'an*, trans. Cheng Chien Bhikshu. (Jain Publishing Co., 1992).

6. Carré, *Huang Po, Maître Tch'an du IXème siècle*. English translation here by Clare Frock.

7. D. T. Suzuki, trans., *The Lankavatara Sutra: A Mahayana Text* (Taipei: SMC Publishing, 1991). English translation of the French by Clare Frock.

8. Red Pine, trans., *The Zen Teachings of Bodhidharma* (Berkeley, Calif.: North Point Press, 1984). English translation of the French by Clare Frock.

9. From the Lalita Devi version, published in Daniel Odier, *Le Grand Sommeil des Éveillés* (Gordes: Le Relié, 2000). English translation by Clare Frock.

10. Foyan, *Instant Zen.*

11. Mazu, *Les Entretiens de Mazu.* English translation here by Clare Frock.

12. Hulin, trans., *Le Secret de la déesse Tripura.* English translation here by Clare Frock.

13. English translation of the French from the author's notebooks by Clare Frock.

14. Longchen Rabjam, *The Practice of Dzogchen.* Introduced, translated, and annotated by Tulku Thondup. Ed., Harold Talbott. (Ithaca, N.Y.: Snow Lion Publications, 1989), 364–365.

15. J. C. Cleary and Thomas Cleary, trans./eds., *Zen Letters: The Teachings of Yuanwu*, 67–68.

16. Master Sheng-yen, *Poetry of Enlightenment.* English translation of the French by Clare Frock.

17. English translation of the French from the author's notebooks by Clare Frock.

18. Foyan, *Tch'an Zen.* English translation of the French by Clare Frock.

19. Vimalakirti, *Soutra de la Liberté inconcevable, les enseignements de Vimalakirti.* Trans., Patrick Carré. (Paris: Éditions Fayard, 2000). English translation here by Clare Frock. Complete English translation available by Burton Watson: *Vimalakirti Sutra* (New York: Columbia University Press, 1992).

20. Mazu, *Les entretiens de Mazu.* English translation here by Clare Frock.

21. Kalu Rinpoché, *Le practique de la voie tibétaine.* English translation here by Clare Frock.

22. Master Sheng-yen, *Poetry of Enlightenment*, 39.

23. English translation of the French from the author's notebooks by Clare Frock.

24. English translation of the French from the author's notebooks by Clare Frock.

25. Foyan *Tch'an, Zen.* English translation here by Clare Frock.

26. Chogyam Trungpa, *The Myth of Freedom and the Way of Meditation* (Boston: Shambhala, 1988), 157–163.

Conclusion

1. For more details on the practice and other texts and references, see the Web site www.danielodier.com.

2. From the oral teachings of the author's master, Lalita Devi.

3. *Dakini Teachings: Padmasambhava's Oral Instructions to Lady Tsogyal*, Recorded and concealed by Yeshe Tsogyal. Revealed by Nyang Ral Nyima Oser and Sangye Lingpa. Translated by Erik Pema Kunsang. (Boston: Shambhala, 1990), page reference unfound. English translation of the author's French by Clare Frock. See note at end of citation for page references of the passages that follow.

4. *Dakini Teachings,* 153 and 56–57.

Appendix 1

1. From Daniel Odier, *Tantra Yoga: le Vijnanabhairava tantra* (Paris: Albin Michel, 1998 and 2004). Translation and commentary by Daniel Odier. English translation by Jeanric Meller.

Appendix 2

1. From *Essential Tibetan Buddhism*, Robert A. F. Thurman (New York: HarperSan Francisco, 1995), 261–264.

BOOKS OF RELATED INTEREST

Tantric Kali
Secret Practices and Rituals
by Daniel Odier

Tantric Quest
An Encounter with Absolute Love
by Daniel Odier

The Heart of Yoga
Developing a Personal Practice
by T. K. V. Desikachar

The Path of Modern Yoga
The History of an Embodied Spiritual Practice
by Elliott Goldberg

The Practice of Nada Yoga
Meditation on the Inner Sacred Sound
by Baird Hersey
Foreword by Sri Krishna Das

Yoga of the Mahamudra
The Mystical Way of Balance
by Will Johnson

Chakras
Energy Centers of Transformation
by Harish Johari

Tools for Tantra
by Harish Johari

Inner Traditions • Bear & Company
P.O. Box 388
Rochester, VT 05767
1-800-246-8648
www.InnerTraditions.com

Or contact your local bookseller